"So often when trying to diets. This book can help y through an easy, healthy w~~ ~~

—Courtney Cox, actress, star of "Friends"

"FEELING LIGHT is a healthy, balanced approach to weight loss."

—Michael Tierra, OMD, author of
The Way of Herbs and *Planetary Herbology*

"This interestingly-written book provides several insightful and innovative components of a comprehensive life-long weight management program."

—Dr. Joseph E. Pizzorno, Jr., ND,
President, Bastyr University

"FEELING LIGHT provides an easy-to-read, up-to-date progressive approach to achieving and maintaining weight loss while maximizing optimum health. A must for any health practitioner treating weight management or anyone interested in losing weight and keeping it off."

—Dr. Allan Magaziner, D.O., M.D.,
Magaziner Medical Center, Cherry Hill, NJ

"Shoshanna and Wendy are throwing away your scales and helping you get in touch with your body's wisdom. By integrating Eastern and Western knowledge, you will obtain satisfaction of mind, body and spirit. This is a practical guide to a new way of life, where you will truly feel lighter."

—Dr. Marianne Roosels, M.D.,
Internal Medicine, Shrewsbury, NJ

"As a pharmacist I know the traditional methods of weight loss have not worked . . . the only true solution is a method like FEELING LIGHT that encompasses life-style changes that can be successful and permanent."

—William Statter, P.D.

"At long last, I have found a book about weight loss that I can recommend to women. Shoshanna Katzman and Wendy Shankin-Cohen offer women a revolutionary vision that is, at its core, about balance, wellness, and ultimately, power."

—Jacqueline Hudak, M.Ed., Family Therapist

"Katzman and Shankin-Cohen present an inspiring program for making healthful and lasting changes in our lives. Their focus on the whole person and steady yet flexible practice offers a balanced approach to nutrition and well-being."

—David A. Landy, Ph.D., Psychologist

"Following these guidelines, one can, with surprising ease, enter a conscious and holistic relationship with one's body where the outcome is truly feeling light."

—Judy Krusell, Ph.D., Psychologist and
Energy Healing Practitionist

"This book is a product of knowledgeable and caring professionals who are clearly dedicated to encouraging their readers up the path of good health and wellness. I highly recommend it to colleagues and students."

—Barbara Lee Rosoff, Ph.D.,
Educator and author, Rumson, NJ

FEELING LIGHT

The Holistic Solution
to Permanent Weight Loss
and Wellness

SHOSHANNA KATZMAN AND **WENDY SHANKIN-COHEN**
WITH **MELINDA MARSHALL**

AVON BOOKS ◆ NEW YORK

The authors do not directly or indirectly dispense medical advice or prescribe the use of diet as a form of treatment for sickness without medical approval. Nutritionists and other experts in the field of health and nutrition hold widely varying views. It is not the intent of the authors to diagnose or prescribe. This book is not meant to be an individualized course of treatment and the reader should consult his or her own qualified health practitioner before engaging in any diet plan. In the event you use the information in this book without your health care provider's approval, you are prescribing for yourself, which is your constitutional right, but the publisher and authors assume no responsibility.

AVON BOOKS
A division of
The Hearst Corporation
1350 Avenue of the Americas
New York, New York 10019

Copyright © 1997 by Shoshanna Katzman, Wendy Shankin-Cohen, and Melinda Marshall
Front cover art by Artemis Design
Published by arrangement with the authors
Visit our website at http://AvonBooks.com
Library of Congress Catalog Card Number: 96-36827
ISBN: 0-380-79097-1

Library of Congress Cataloging in Publication Data:
Katzman, Shoshanna.
    Feeling light : the holistic solution to permanent weight loss and wellness / Shoshanna Katzman and Wendy Shankin-Cohen with Melinda Marshall.
        p.   cm.
    1. Weight loss.   2. Health.   3. Holistic medicine.   I. Shankin-Cohen, Wendy.
    II. Marshall, Melinda M., 1961–   .   III. Title.
RM222.2.K365   1997   96-36827
613.2'5—dc21   CIP

First Avon Books Trade Printing: February 1997

AVON TRADEMARK REG. U.S. PAT. OFF. AND IN OTHER COUNTRIES, MARCA REGISTRADA, HECHO EN U.S.A.

Printed in the U.S.A.

OPM 10 9 8 7 6 5 4 3 2 1

We dedicate this book to those who didn't believe they could, those who didn't know how, and those who have found the courage to seek balance in their lives to heal themselves, their families, and our planet.

From Wendy: To my mother who has always been my inspiration. Who with incredible balance, grace, courage, and love taught me to reach high but stay centered. No child could receive a greater gift. To my Pop who has become a force in my life, a true guide and source of support and love. To my children, Ty, Remy, and Lincoln, who are the joy. And to my husband, Dr. Harvey Cohen, whose knowledge of how to give to others taught me "all I need to know."

From Shoshanna: To my dearest husband, Michael, who has provided endless support and encouragement. To my daughter Hilary, for being so understanding, and my sons, Noah and Jared, for loving their mommy unconditionally. To my wonderful in-laws, Shirlee and Aaron, for their love and support. And to my parents, Marilyn and Abe, who have taught me through example—patience, understanding, love for life, and an insatiable quest for knowledge.

ACKNOWLEDGMENTS

Shoshanna and Wendy wish to thank those who have given knowledge, support, time, love and who have helped the dream become a reality: Jeff Breedlove, Richard Brenner, Sal Canizzaro, Harvey Cohen, D.C., Roger and Janice Colley, Subhuti Dharmananda, Ph.D., Patricia Early, Fong Ha, Sarah Hall, Bing Jiang, Larry Johnson, O.M.D., Nancy Kahan, Ted Kaptchuk, O.M.D., Michael Katzman, Philip Lansky, M.D., Miriam Lee, O.M.D., Shawna McCarthy, Debra McGuire, Marcy and Brian McMullen, Dahlia Reid, Holly Roberts, D.O., Sonia Rodd, Marianne Roosels, M.D., Vega Rosenberg, Madelyne and Edward Ryterband, Ph.D., Danny Sanchez, Kerry Savage, Mark Seems, Ph.D., Bruce Shankin, Johanna Stavrou, Michael Tierra, O.M.D., Kelly Van Sickell, C.A., Barbara Zebora, Christine Zika, Shoshanna's Tai Chi students, five sisters and brothers-in-law, all of our Feeling Light participants, clients, and patients, and most especially Melinda Marshall, whose "genius without ego" is a truly rare find, as she has made this process a dream within a dream.

ABOUT THE AUTHORS

SHOSHANNA KATZMAN, C.A., M.A.

Ms. Katzman is an acupuncturist, Chinese herbalist, and Tai Chi master. She received her Masters Degree in Sports Medicine from San Francisco State University in 1981. She is a 1984 graduate of a California state approved Acupuncture Tutorial Program under the direction of Michael Tierra, OMD and Miriam Lee, OMD, and a 1987 graduate of the Tristate Institute of Traditional Chinese Acupuncture. She has been the director of the Red Bank Acupuncture and Wellness Center in New Jersey since 1987.

Ms. Katzman has been a practicing acupuncturist since 1984 and is nationally certified by the National Commission for the Certification of Acupuncturists (NCCA) and state board certified in California, Maryland, New Jersey, New York, and Pennsylvania. She has been a practitioner and teacher of Tai Chi Chuan and Chi Gong exercise since 1974. She is the founder of two martial arts schools, one in Santa Cruz, California, the other in Red Bank, New Jersey.

Ms. Katzman is married and is the mother of three children.

WENDY SHANKIN-COHEN, M.F.A.

Ms. Shankin-Cohen is the director of Holistic Health Consultants located in Red Bank, New Jersey, and is a private consultant specializing in Homeopathic Education and Holistic Nutrition. She is the educator for one of the largest homeopathic study groups in the United States and a member of the National Center for Homeopathy.

Ms. Shankin-Cohen earned a B.A. from the University of Michigan in 1972 and an M.F.A. at New York University in 1976. Ms. Shankin-Cohen is the mother of three sons and along with her husband Dr. Harvey Cohen, a pioneer of natural health for animals. She continues to teach and lecture throughout the United States.

About the Feeling Light Program

The Feeling Light Program is an inspirational, motivational, experiential, and informative two-hour session that meets weekly in Little Silver, New Jersey. These sessions provide the opportunity for the participants to experience firsthand the techniques described in this book. The two-hour session begins with bellows breathing exercises and stretching and then moves into Tai Chi. The participants are then seated and receive acupuncture along with instruction and practice of self-acupressure. During the acupuncture session the group is led in a guided meditation. A general discussion follows on supplementation, nutrition, herbs, flower essences, recipes, and personal stories about how to integrate Feeling Light into one's life. A variety of other topics are discussed, including mindful eating and living, cardiovascular exercise and weight training, how to travel Feeling Light, and food combining. Participants also learn to prepare and have a chance to taste the healthful and delicious Feeling Light Recipes.

Plans are underway to open Feeling Light Centers throughout North America. For more information on Feeling Light Programs, please call toll free 888–222–8400 or write to Feeling Light, c/o Healthquest, P.O. Box 8723, Red Bank, NJ 07701.

CONTENTS

FEELING LIGHT

Are You Ready for a Transformation?

Maybe you're new at this. Maybe you've never worried about your weight, questioned your diet, or suffered from any sort of chronic ailment. Maybe the extra pounds have snuck up on you in your sleep, along with age spots and spider veins, and now you're suddenly keen on reversing the decline.

But if you're overweight, chances are you're a seasoned player in the weight loss game, and you're mighty leery of anyone promising any kind of "transformation." You've embraced the latest "breakthrough" more than once, after all. You've gone on regimens of sardines and cheese, grapefruit and eggs, cottage cheese and lean meat. You've counted calories, carbohydrates, and grams of fat. You've popped pills, sprinkled on powders, and mixed up milk shakes. You've cut down on fat and protein and loaded up on pasta and vegetables, until the next medical expert prescribed low carbs and high protein, and a formerly overweight housewife determined you were likely allergic to carbohydrates and recommended cutting them out altogether. You've been to group meetings. You've bought prepackaged foods. You may have even sold vitamins or powders.

Not that these diets didn't transform you. A lot of them did—briefly. It's just that now you're back where you started, only a little heavier, a little more tired, a little more defeated, and a lot more skeptical. Because all those diet doctors, former fatties, liquid protein manufacturers, and health gurus profited hugely from your sporadic losses.

We've counseled hundreds of people over the past decade, and even those who manage to stick to the Standard American Diet (S.A.D., appropriately enough) feel betrayed. They're not only overweight, many of them: they're not well. They feel lousy. They're riddled with a host of complaints, from irritable bowel syndrome and high blood pressure to degenerative diseases like atherosclerosis and osteoporosis. Many complain of chronic fatigue. More than a few are on antidepressants. They seek us out to help them make a change because their health—even their lives—depends on a transformation. Losing weight is not always at the top of their list.

But in the course of getting our clients well, a funny thing happens. Those who were feeling depressed feel a terrible weight lifting. Those who were stricken with exhaustion find their energies restored. And those who were overweight start shedding the pounds.

Feeling better, for many of our patients, has translated into feeling spiritually invigorated. Mentally rejuvenated. Physically buoyant. In a word, they feel *lighter*.

WHAT IS HOLISTIC WEIGHT MANAGEMENT?

Feeling Light™ is a weight management program that has evolved from the real-life experiences of those who've come to us over the years seeking better health. We're not academicians who postulated what should work, theoretically, and then waited for someone to prove us right. We started with an observation: excess weight, like any other physical complaint, is merely a symptom, a red flag signaling inner illness and pointing to a fundamental imbalance of vital energies. Address that inner imbalance, and all outward manifestations of illness—weight included—disappear.

Hence holistic weight management is simply an outgrowth of our holistic approach to health, which is to heal mind, body, and soul rather than offer purely symptomatic relief. We use herbs, nutritional supplements, accupressure and acupuncture tailored to correct each individual's specific imbalance. And we suggest dietary changes to speed the healing process—cutting down on animal protein, dairy, and sugar, loading up on fruits, vegetables, and whole grains.

So what's revolutionary about this program? The fact that weight loss isn't the focus. It's more like a perk—one of many—you get when you subscribe to our plan for better health. Make no mistake: Feeling Light is a health plan, not a diet. There's no deprivation, no forbidden foods, no weird food combinations or stringent eating timetables. We don't count calories or measure portions. We don't tally pounds lost or inches pinched. And we don't ever use guilt as a form of dietary discipline.

*   *   *

Participants in our weekly Feeling Light workshop continue to marvel that we don't talk about weight for the two-plus hours we spend together. Many of them report that this is the first group program they actually look forward to attending, even to the point where they'll cancel other meetings and events. For them, Feeling Light is an oasis of relaxation, gentle exercise, and fun learning in an otherwise relentless workweek.

For you, we've distilled out of the workshop everything you need to start your own healing process. As with our class, we've tried to structure this book so that you can feel comfortable dropping in at any point, for any length of time. You can start at the beginning, or zero in on our discussion of the yin-yang food gradient, or even join us at the conclusion, where we lay out daily, weekly, monthly, and seasonal game plans for health—and then you can work backward as you like.

This isn't a two-week crash program or a weekend indoctrination, however. Feeling Light is going to change the way you think about food, the way you eat, and the way you see the world; such dramatic changes take place successfully only if they take place gradually. Transformation doesn't happen overnight; it's a journey undertaken for the journey itself, not the destination. Weight loss is but one sign of progress.

Our clients do, however, almost universally start *feeling* better—more energetic, less depressed, better able to cope—*immediately*. And some report even losing upwards of a pound a week.

WILL IT WORK FOR ME?

Those who've attended the Feeling Light workshops have come from every walk of life, lifestyle, and outlook. Some have dieted all their lives and want to get off the fad treadmill of the diet industry. Some, worn to a frazzle by the workaday world, come looking for stress management. Others can't specify what they're looking for, except to feel better.

They come willingly, and hopefully—but not without reservations. Feeling Light, after all, is like nothing they've ever tried. We know that. In all likelihood, their reservations echo your own. We can't effect a transformation if you're burdened with doubts or anxieties, so before we promise you a transforming experience, let's clear up any misunderstandings. Here are the concerns we hear aired most frequently:

I've tried every diet and weight management program out there that guarantees rapid weight loss. They're all hype.
We're inclined to agree. Radical changes require radical tactics—and life is too multifaceted to make significant changes overnight. When we open our Thursday night class with the reminder that Feeling Light is a ten-year program, there's an audible sigh of relief. Everyone knows from bitter experience that trying to meet some unreasonable "deadline" for weight loss exerts the kind of pressure that guarantees failure.

I've always succeeded in losing weight—it's just that it always comes back.
You're not alone. A recent government study found that only 1 out of every 200 adults who tries to lose weight succeeds in taking off and keeping off 10 pounds or more a year later. Any program that promises you'll lose weight if you temporarily put aside your normal dietary habits is just that: temporary. Feeling Light will make you conscious of what you choose to put in your mouth for the rest of your life.

I'm too depressed to go on a diet.
Depression is one of the most often cited reasons people seek out our help. They may be overweight, they may be depressed about

*being overweight, or—as is typically the case—their body chem-
istry and equilibrium are so out of whack they simply feel lousy,
depressed, and fat. We address that inner illness holistically,
with proper nutrition, flower essences, nutritional supplements,
breathing exercises called chi gong, bellows breathing, energizing movements called Tai Chi, acupuncture, acupressure, and
meditation. By healing the body from the inside out, outward
symptoms such as depression and unwanted weight disappear
with the imbalance that caused them.*

I'm not into meditation or any of that New Age stuff.
*We're not going to try and sell you crystals. We don't live in
an ashram, and we don't expect you to drop out of the Western
world in order to get healthy or lose weight. Many of our participants were skeptical of the meditative exercises we showed
them; most of them have found, however, that at the very least
meditation enforces a peace that brings relaxation. We urge
everyone to practice certain affirmations daily, because we've observed that these positive statements work whether you believe
in them or not. We believe in the power of the mind to heal the
body, but we've seen it work the other way around, too.*

I don't have time to eat right.
*Too many of us respond to the pressures of work, family, and
modern life by whirling like a dervish. Everything is important,
everything must get done today, right this minute. We're so
needled by guilt and fear that we can't sit down for even a moment, even if it's for something as vital as eating.*

*We can't add a twenty-fifth or twenty-sixth hour to your
day, but we can help you insist on taking the time to sit down,
calm down, and nourish your whole self. Not surprisingly, people who eat right feel better, and those who feel better cope better.
Eating harmful foods, on the other hand, skews inner equilibrium
and leaves one vulnerable to panic attacks and panic eating. Our
clients report that a cup of hot water with a calming essence can*

be enough to silence the nagging and self-defeating "hurry-up"
voice that can sabotage sensible eating.

**I know when I'm eating the wrong food. It's just that I
can't help myself.**
*A craving for non-nourishing food is like a scab: it itches, you
scratch it—even though you know you're getting in the way of
the healing process. So you eat poorly, conscious only that you're
hungering for something. Unhealthy foods exaggerate the imbalance that gives rise to cravings, leaving you helpless to stop
wanting. That's the vicious cycle dooming most dieters to failure.
If the body's sick, it's in no shape to dictate its own cure.*

*That's why we start with the mind. We arm our clients with
a list of simple but effective affirmations to recite in times of
crisis. With flower essences, we help them reach a state of inner
peace; with meditation, we can help them strengthen inner resolve. And then, because unchecked cravings can cause such
physical torment, we use acupuncture and acupressure to quell
those desires at their source. That gives the body a fighting
chance, because once our clients regain nutritional balance, they
find they no longer crave unhealthy foods.*

**I don't see how I could stand acupuncture. Even thinking
about needles makes me feel uptight.**
*Funny thing about that: ask anybody who's received treatment,
and almost universally they'll report on how relaxing they
found it. The ancients were not any more tolerant of pain than
we are, and they would have questioned a practice that hurt in
order to heal. If you're really squeamish, however, acupressure
can prove to be an effective alternative.*

**I can't fast. I've tried, and I never make it. I start craving
like crazy and then I eat even more than I would have.**
*Fasting is a scary prospect for most people. Because it has cus-
tomarily been the dieter's gotta-lose-five-pounds-by-tomorrow*

last resort, we associate fasting with the worst kind of deprivation, and we fret about our ability to endure. Just as most of us
would not attempt to run a marathon without training for it,
we're not about to subject ourselves to a test for which we're not
mentally and physically conditioned.

Well, there's no endurance testing in our program. But we
are going to condition you for what we term a cleansing fast,
and when you feel ready, you can begin. The idea is not to lose
weight (although you will) but rather to flush out all the toxins
clinging to your intestinal tract and impairing absorption of
foods that can start the healing process. You choose the fast you
feel up to—brown rice and veggies, or fruit, or just juice or
water—and the duration. But because we give you the tools to
squelch hunger, even the most fast-resistant of our clients find
they feel absolutely fine—light!—during their detoxification.

I don't want to lose weight. I'd just like to eat better.
Lose, gain, or stay the same—whatever your goal, Feeling Light
can help you get there by showing you how different kinds of
food affect your mind/body equilibrium. If you're out of kilter
because you've been eating at the extremes, you'll learn how to
counter the effects and get closer to the middle, where true balance—and optimal health—lie.

Feeling Light isn't just a weapon against weight disorders.
Eating a holistically balanced diet is your best defense against
degenerative diseases and terminal illness. Studies from the medical community on the healthful effects of a diet high in fiber and
antioxidants simply confirm what some cultures have known—
and practiced—for centuries.

**How can I get enough protein and calcium if I don't eat
any meat or dairy products?**
Fifty years of being bombarded with propaganda from the beef
and dairy industries would leave anyone a trifle concerned about
cutting out animal protein or by-products. But it's no coinci-

dence that Americans have the most protein- and calcium-rich diet in the world—and one of the highest rates of heart disease and osteoporosis. If meat were essential, billions of vegetarians over the past two millennia would surely have figured that out by now. If dairy were essential, then why are so many people lactose-intolerant?

This all sounds too good to be true.
If we suggested we could change the way you eat, the way you treat your body, and the way you see yourself in the world in a matter of weeks, you'd be absolutely right: too good to be true. So take a look again at our contents page, because what we're offering is not the Holy Grail but a road map toward total mind/ body health. How closely you stick to the route and how fast you go are entirely up to you.

*You may be at a point in your life where you're utterly receptive to change and ready to prioritize your own health; you may, on the other hand, be gradually working toward the realization that wellness is an investment you need to make now if you want to avoid bankruptcy down the line. We're here to help you make that change, to show you the way toward optimal health and weight management. We're here to make the journey comfortable, even fun. The healing process may take some time, but we can assure you you'll feel better—*lighter *in mind, body, and spirit—almost immediately.*

If that *sounds too good to be true, then read on.*

PART ONE

Get Ready...

CHAPTER ONE

The Mind/Body Approach to Weight Management

*We must change direction
or we will end up where we are headed.*
—Chinese proverb

All diets work.

Really. You can bet that for every bit of wacko dieting wisdom out there, somewhere there is someone who at some time lost some weight by taking that wisdom to heart. No carbohydrates for two weeks? Sure. Jenny Craig frozen entrees for two months? Okay. Forty percent protein, 30 percent carbohydrates, and 30 percent monounsaturated fats every meal? Probably works, if you're a chemist.

All diets work, which is to say you'll lose weight while you're on them. Even a lot of weight. But then what? Say you've adopted the latest all-protein regimen. Say you've dropped fourteen pounds in as many days. Say you're happy with your new weight. Now the big question: are you going to keep eating this way?

Better not. Every piece of research conducted over the last twenty years by everyone from nutritionists to nephrologists, from the U.S. Department of Health and Human Services to Harvard Medical School, underscores the correlation between diets low in fiber (low in fruits and vegetables) and high in fat (high in animal and dairy products) and the six major killers in this country—cancer, stroke, heart disease, atherosclerosis, diabetes . . . and obesity. A diet consisting of mostly protein is invariably a diet of meat, fish, and dairy, because few other foods offer a comparable concentration of protein. Chances are, if you're making protein the predominant source of your calories, you're probably getting plenty of fat and cholesterol, too, and nowhere near enough dietary fiber. You're also missing out on the cancer-fighting phytochemicals and antioxidants that vegetables, fruits, and grains provide—insurance you could really use, because animal products these days are laced with hormones, pesticide residue, heavy metals, and antibiotics.

Add to this argument the fact that excessive protein leaches vital minerals from your bones and tissues, putting a toxic load on your kidneys and setting you up for osteoporosis, and you've got a diet that provides short-term weight loss at the cost of long-term health. Which is the trade-off that every diet since the refinement of sugar has asked you to weigh: your waistline or your life. Your weight or your health. The way you look, or the way you feel and function.

No, wait just a minute, you're shaking your head. *I'm dieting to get healthy! That's what everyone's been telling me: If I don't lose the weight, I'll lose my health.*

Ah. Glad you brought that up. Because this is what years of experience have proven to us repeatedly: You have a weight problem *because* you're not well. You're not in balance. In fact, *you won't lose weight* unless *you get healthy.* And dieting is no way to nourish your body back to a state of well-being.

NEVER SAY DIET

Diets win you battles but lose you the war. They work, and then they don't work, because all the while you're reaping results you're sowing the seeds of your undoing. They undermine you at the most fundamental of levels, conning you into believing that your body is an enemy, an unruly child to be disciplined, punished, constantly denied. A diet asks you to see yourself as two separate entities: the half that's in charge (the mind) and the half that's out of control (the body). The typical diet book takes the disciplinarian in you aside and says, "You've let this child of yours get way out of hand. Now it's time to get tough. It's time to lay down the law. From now on, the kid gets no more _____" (you fill in the blank).

The disciplinarian nods. The body rebels. And so continues the endless cycle of punishment and indulgence, diet and weight gain. Every time the scale reads a higher number, the child is rebuked and denied certain pleasures. The child is put on a diet. The child dutifully performs under scrutiny, all the while biding his time for the next opportunity to disobey.

This kind of power struggle never works—not in child-rearing, and not in weight management. A child who acts out is really crying for comfort and attention; a body that won't "behave" in its eating habits is likewise crying out for nourishment and nurturing. A child denied love doesn't learn to stop needing it; a body denied the foods it craves only intensifies its search. A child who's told repeatedly he's not good enough will eventually stop trying to be good; a body admonished repeatedly that it's not thin enough will ultimately balloon up with weight until the mind feels the despair of total failure.

If you want to set yourself up for this kind of failure— over and over—then you'll adopt the dieter's image of mind and body in constant struggle.

If you're ready for a new tactic—if you're ready for Feeling Light—you'll stop seeing yourself this way. You'll stop fighting yourself. You'll stop pitting allies against each other.

Parent and child, mind and body, are one and the same. This isn't just New Age–speak: Candace Pert, a Georgetown University biochemistry professor, actually quantified it, showing how brain and body communicate using a network of chemical messengers called peptides. According to Pert, these peptides are the "biochemical units of emotion" because they translate our every thought, reaction, and emotion into physiological change. Our organs, tissue, skin, muscle, and endocrine glands all have peptide receptors on them and can store, access, and "act" upon emotional information. "Thoughts" or "feelings" may not only affect, say, the operation of the digestive organs; they may, in all likelihood, *originate* in those organs. This means that conceptualizing mind as the seat of emotional memory is a false conception: memory is a string of protein molecules that can be stored in the tissues of the pancreas just as easily as in the nerve cells of the brain. Of course, Pert, former chief of the section on brain biochemistry at the National Institutes of Health, has simply validated with Western science what Eastern philosophies established millennia ago: the mind is literally the body.

So this false division between them—a division encouraged by the diet industry—must be healed. You must take that child you've been punishing and embrace him as a precious and dear part of you. No more denial. No more divisive tactics. Mind and body are on your side. They're in this lifelong journey of yours together, wedded at the cellular level, incapable of acting independently of each other. You are what you believe, you do what you think, and you manifest what you feel. Your biography, as Deepak Chopra has written, becomes your biology. An overweight or underweight physique is simply the sculpture cast by emotional turmoil, unvented stress, biochemical chaos. A body with a weight problem is a mind/body that's imbalanced, that's ailing, that's in need of overall *healing*.

HOW TO BEGIN THE HEALING PROCESS

Throw out your scale.

That's one of the first things we tell our Feeling Light participants, because most of them have had a scale attached to the soles of their feet most of their lives, and it has weighed on them like a ball and chain. They'd like to be rid of the thing, but then they just don't know themselves without it. It's a measurement they must have of themselves. It's like the parent, externalized: the numbers can be gold stars for excellent behavior or black marks for disobedience.

Some of our clients won't part with this parent. Their self-image is charted by the numbers they see displayed there. Weight in our culture has come to represent who will be desirable and worthy and who will not, so the bathroom scale offers a daily measurement of self-worth. But then it has the power to make or break our day, to set us up for the failure/success seesaw. It has the power to make us launch an all-out assault against ourselves. It has the

power to convince us we are what we weigh, and we are
worth what we look like.

> Feeling Light *is* concerned with how you look. But
> more importantly, Feeling Light is concerned with
> how you feel: Do you feel well? Do you feel good?
> Do you feel good about yourself?

Those are the appropriate questions to ask each morning, in lieu of stepping up for moral judgment. The last
thing you need when you're chronically ailing is a guilt
trip; guilt is one of the many emotions that gets you to eat,
not to refrain from eating. Nor do you need another reason
for self-flagellation; hating yourself and your body is part
of the reason you overeat. In our personal experience, and
in the experience of those we've helped lose weight, the
worst motivators are guilt ("I'm not perfect and I screwed
up"); fear ("If I don't lose weight, I'm going to be unlov-
able and live a short, unhappy life"); and competition
("Mary lost a pound a day on this diet; why can't I?").
We want to take the focus off your weight because
Feeling Light is about your health—about first and foremost *getting you well*. For that, you won't need a scale to
see if you're making progress. You'll know you are, because you'll feel it, and you'll see it. You'll feel it in your
bones, you'll see it in your skin. You'll feel it in your outlook, in the way you wear your clothes, in the way you
bound out of bed, in the way you greet each day and each
new challenge. And each day, you'll feel better than the
day before. Isn't this how getting healthy *should* feel? Isn't
this how losing weight should feel?
Your body is the only vehicle you'll get to buoy you
through this life. Its shape or size, however unwieldy, is
not a betrayal of your wishes, but a plea for your attention—for your caring, your nurturing, your healing, and

your daily maintenance. If you feel bloated, tired, draggy, depressed, sluggish, or thick, it's because you're not well. And when you're sick, you need to care for yourself, not go on some diet that makes you feel even worse. Stop looking at your weight as something obscuring the perfect you, something hanging on you like a bad suit. Fat is an outgrowth of inner imbalance. Imbalance is what we're here to address.

> ## —THE PHYSIOLOGY OF BEHAVIOR—
>
> People eat too much, too little, or too poorly out of an unanswered, insatiable *need*.

It's possible that this need arises from a vitamin or mineral deficiency, an inadequate fatty acid intake, an overworked liver, or a wildly spiking and dropping blood sugar level. It's possible this need stems from an emotional cause: an abusive marriage, a troubled childhood, an alcoholic family member. It's possible that this need points to a spiritual void, one that food seems to fill in the absence of a belief system.

It's entirely probable that this need, this weight problem, this drive to eat and eat badly, is the outgrowth of *all* these factors—physical, emotional, and spiritual imbalances. They're all interrelated. They must all be addressed, simultaneously. That's what Feeling Light does, which no other "diet" can do: it works holistically. It's as thorough as the problem of weight is pervasive.

But to understand why you need our holistic approach, first you've got to understand how mind, body, and mouth work on each other's feedback.

Let's begin with blood sugar. Blood sugar levels are all

the buzz in diet circles right now, as if hypoglycemia were a disease and as if it were epidemic in America. And indeed, it does seem that way: client after client has come to us insisting that they suffer from blood sugar crashes that compel them to eat.

As a clinical diagnosis, hypoglycemia describes a condition in which glucose, or blood sugar, dips drastically *for no apparent reason*. We say no apparent reason, because there are plenty of really good reasons why blood sugar plunges. For instance, just about everybody has experienced hypoglycemic episodes by eating a lot of sugar or other simple carbohydrate, thereby jacking up blood sugar levels so high, so fast, that there's no place else to go but down—real low, real fast. It's easy to induce these spikes: just about everything on the supermarket shelves these days is made from carbohydrates that have been simplified—stripped of their original nutrients—through the refining process. Vitamins and minerals that would normally slow down the body's absorption rate, tempering the release of sugar into the bloodstream, are absent. Simple sugars are thus absorbed hyper-fast, sending blood sugar levels soaring soon after ingestion. Some of the foods likeliest to trigger a hypoglycemic episode, ironically enough, are those labeled "fat-free," because high fructose corn syrup, sugar, fructose, and dextrose make up for the fats that have been taken out.

The reason blood sugar plunges to levels below normal—hypoglycemia—after shooting sky-high has to do with something called insulin response. Insulin is a hormone secreted by the pancreas to help ferry glucose from the blood into the cells, which "eat" glucose as fuel. How quickly the pancreas releases insulin to deal with sugar-saturated blood depends on the individual; some individuals, after bombarding their systems with sweets, experience an insulin "delay." For some reason, the pancreas fails to notice a rise in blood sugar until levels are toxic, and then it overcompensates with too much insulin. Insulin hustles glucose into the cells so thoroughly and so fast that there's a sudden deficit in blood sugar. The individual feels shaky, weak, irritable . . . and driven to replace the sugar his bloodstream now lacks.

It's almost as if one's cells, after getting a massive jolt of glucose, become greedy for more. That's the cycle refined sugars induce: the more you get, the more you want. Soon after a sugary meal, it seems, you get a vicious "hunger" attack. Except that the more you ingest, the more sluggishly your insulin responds, much as a horse repeatedly spurred slows down rather than speeds up. In some people, the condition becomes irreversible: they're termed diabetic, because insulin production is so deficient or unresponsive that blood sugar remains high while the cells literally starve to death.

So when our clients term themselves "hypoglycemic," it's not that we doubt they experience debilitating blood sugar lows that compel them to eat. They most surely do. But we suspect that their eating habits are to blame for this "insulin resistance" or "carbohydrate sensitivity," as the diet industry now calls this vicious cycle. Some individuals are indeed born with a pancreas that doesn't regulate the production or release of insulin very well; our bet is that many Americans *condition* their pancreases into sluggishness, by repeatedly flooding their systems with sugars that cannot be processed moderately.

A steady diet of soda, crackers, cookies, candy, juice drinks, white flour pasta, white flour bread, sugary cereal, and "fat-free" desserts is bound to affect insulin response. Over time, under a constant barrage of nutritionally stripped carbohydrates, the pancreas responds with ill-timed, ill-measured insulin secretion *no matter what* food is ingested. If thousands of Americans are warming to the idea that they're "insulin resistant" or "carbohydrate-sensitive," it's not because Americans are born any different from the rest of the world, but because they most certainly eat differently from the rest of the world, beginning at birth with a formula of corn syrup solids. It is no coincidence that Type II diabetes (diabetes mellitus) is more common here than in any other country.

THE LIVER'S ROLE IN OBESITY

Insulin response to carbohydrates is not the only factor in hypoglycemia and obesity. In some people, the liver is just not doing its job. And again, these people were not born with a second-rate liver; they acquired it through dietary habit.

Overeating or eating overly refined foods whose nutritional value has been compromised overworks the liver. An overworked liver is one that can't do its job of sending nutrients to the cells and storing excess glucose. An overworked liver allows too much sugar into the bloodstream and too many toxins into the blood and brain. This biochemical "poisoning," in turn, triggers the release or suppression of any number of other hormones and brain chemicals responsible for emotional well-being. Adrenaline, for example, keeps flooding the system in response to low blood sugar, leaving in its wake a gnawing anxiety, agitation, and a sense of imminent emergency. Except, there's no real emergency here. No dragon to slay, no enemy to run from—just a low blood sugar attack from eating an entire box of SnackWell's Double Truffles.

Our hypoglycemic client rightly describes this feeling as *lousy*. Shaky. Frantic. Irritable. Like she needs to *do* something, but just can't. Like she *needs* something, but just can't put a finger on it. (Though she'll try, by sampling everything in the refrigerator, the kitchen cupboards, or the office vending machine.) Add to this adrenaline-induced mania the depression caused by a polluted central nervous system and you've got a physical/emotional disaster. You've got someone physiologically and psychologically driven to find relief in food.

Hence the mind/body/mouth circuit goes something like this: You eat bad food, which is to say, you eat the standard American diet of white flour, white sugar, refined salt, and saturated animal fats. You pollute or overload your liver to the point where it can't keep contaminants from entering the bloodstream, and it can't regulate blood sugar levels. You put excessive demand on your pancreas to produce insulin, until insulin response is all out of whack. The resultant hypoglycemia spurs the release of adrenaline, creating a stressful stew of emotions and an eating attack. You eat more, but you get less satisfaction out of it because your neurotransmitters aren't getting the nutrients they need to manufacture the chemicals that would normally send out a signal to STOP.

You're not getting the message anymore. The messenger has been bound and gagged. Mind and body, which normally operate as a beautifully synchronized unit, cannot understand or respond to their own communication. You're a house divided. Your body is now the enemy—the child who won't listen. And the mind/disciplinarian is on the brink of despair.

—HEALING THE MIND/BODY SCHISM—

The answer is balance.

Feeling Light offers an alternative, a set of tools designed to reintegrate mind and body so that you're not fighting yourself anymore. These tools are laid out by chapter, and while you can pick and choose, experience has proven to us the value of bringing them all to bear. They work best together. We believe a holistic approach is the only approach to weight management, given the deep-seated nature of imbalance.

And your weight problem will vanish, but don't fixate on it. Weight loss is only one of the signs that you're recovering from years of abusive conditioning. You've got to open yourself up to the big picture. The picture you see in that little window where you read the numbers on your scale is much too confined, much too simplistic a view. The weight "problem" you see there is, if you raise your perspective, a symptom, merely; the diet you would normally choose ("lose a pound a day!") is but a Band-Aid for that symptom. You're dying to lose weight, and that's exactly why you're not succeeding: you're literally compromising your health when you adopt one of those diets. As we've said, throw out your scale, and you'll be forced to notice things that signal wellness other than weight. Energy levels, sleep patterns, coping skills, tastes in food, changes in cravings, attitudes toward change or challenge, elasticity in skin tone, muscular flexibility, resistance to viral and bacterial infection—these are all perks of Feeling Light.

Bear in mind that curing what ails you deep inside is a process, typically one that takes time, a willingness to learn, and a commitment to change. It won't happen overnight, but neither will it be tortuous and unrewarding along the way. Each step you take, tiny though it may initally seem, will make the next step look that much easier to take. Each result, though it may not be measured in pounds, will help inspire you to stick with the program— to make good, and then better, and then the best, choices. Good choices make you feel better enough to choose the better choices, which in turn speed the healing process such that you're making the best possible choices, over and over, day after day. We know from watching our clients that if only they get to experience a period of wellness, they will keep coming back *of their own free will* to the foods that make them feel that way.

Lynn, 41, is a car wash and pool service owner who, along with her husband, joined Feeling Light to battle a bulge of more than 100 pounds. A few weeks into the program, Lynn says, "We fell into old habits: it just seemed easier to fire up the grill and throw on a few steaks than wash some vegetables or slice up an onion and put that on. Not that it was truly any easier, but when you get emotionally weak, the familiar is what's easiest."

Lynn is no stranger to the power of old habits: she's fought—and overcome—both alcohol and drug addictions. In times of emotional struggle, she turned to food— her solace as well as her remaining self-destructive reflex. When she started slipping from Feeling Light, she says, it was because of emotional crisis—family legal wrangles and the sale of the car wash business. She felt she couldn't cope. She felt like drinking again. She felt like reverting to her old eating habits—and she did.

But then a thought occurred to her: could it be that she felt overwhelmed and unable to cope because she had stopped eating right? Could it be that she was just not dealing with stress well because she didn't feel good? Was it possible that "emotional weakness" wasn't the cause, but the effect, of going off Feeling Light?

"Suddenly, I got it," she says. "When my husband and I were doing the shake (the Feeling Light Smoothie) and the vitamins, and had cut way back on the animal protein, we definitely felt much better. We could deal.

We were so much more positive, not overwhelmed like we're feeling now.

"I realized," she continues, "that if you're out of whack, you can't cope, so you eat more of what makes you unable to cope. When I was doing my meditation, or doing the Tai Chi—when I was taking time for myself—I felt as if I'd rewarded myself. And when I reward myself with those activities, then I don't feel the need to reward myself with food. When I'm doing Feeling Light, I feel good, like I'm doing something positive for myself, like I'm working toward a positive goal. I don't feel like life sucks, who gives a damn; I don't get sucked into that attitude where I think, 'I don't care, so what difference does it make?' I do care. My body and mind appreciate the time I take for myself. I get angry now when I don't take that time, when I don't do the program."

Lynn remembers losing 100 pounds ten years ago and gaining it back, potato chip by potato chip, because the depression she induced convinced her she didn't care, that nothing mattered. In her own words, she "fell off the wagon." She failed.

But there's no such failure possible in Feeling Light. There's bound to be slippage, but no fateful, irreversible relapse. Any deviation from the program is self correcting. Come the holidays, you may succumb to old habits and plow through a plate of cookies, or break down and eat a slab of beef Wellington—but chances are you'll feel so *sick* and awful when you eat "the old way" that you'll feel more committed than ever to Feeling Light. You'll feel you can't wait to cleanse out the damage and start anew. Will you lapse again? Probably, yes—but you won't take but one cookie, and you'll settle on turkey instead of beef. Ultimately, you won't even feel the temptation. You'll have proven to yourself that those former fixations just don't do it for you anymore. They don't deliver satisfaction.

Given the choice, you'll choose health—and it won't feel like sacrifice, it'll feel like a gift. You'll make that choice reflexively, day after day. No more torment. No more guilt. No more "mornings after."

Once you get balanced, you'll enjoy a freedom no diet has ever given you before: You won't have to worry about your weight, obsess about food, or be limited in outlook to the numbers you see displayed in a tiny window at your feet. When your body and mind are healed and once again unified in purpose, food will no longer be an escape, a means of filling empty time, a means of salving emotional wounds, a means of self-destruction. You will look upon eating as an act of caretaking, as both fuel and medicine for the vehicle carrying you through life.

Feeling Light is about changing your *self*. It's about re-uniting your mind and body so that you may see how well mind/body works together, instead of how dramatically it can dysfunction when treated separately. You are not the sum total of your parts. You are not just the size of your waist plus the shape of your thighs. Conventional diets demand that you divide and conquer, that you zero in on fat, on cellulite, as if by eliminating any sign of it you cure yourself of its cause. But you know better, by now. Yank out a weed without its root, and it will grow right back.

If it's a quick, cosmetic fix you're after, then the diet fad-*du-jour* is your best bet—or surgery, or liposuction, or con-trol-top panty hose. If you think the solution is as easy as taking a happy pill, then all too many psychiatrists are ready to accommodate you with a prescription. But if you're ready to see body and mind as one, and if you're ready to acknowledge the holistic nature of the problem,

then Feeling Light offers the only all-encompassing solution. We're here to give you the tools, the instructions, and
the support you need to dig yourself out of the rut you're
likely to bury yourself in. We're here to help you climb
out of it, change direction, and get on the right road. We're
here to make you believe there's a light at the end of the
tunnel—and that you have it within you to reach it and
rejoice in it.

CHAPTER TWO

Readying
the Mind

*In the midst of winter I finally learned
that there was in me an invincible summer.*
                                    —Albert Camus

*R*elax.

How many times have you been told—have you told yourself?—to calm down, chill out, take a deep breath, quit worrying, decompress, or just . . . relax?

Of course you'd *like* to. But you've got things to do, places to rush to, appointments to keep, kids to pick up, bills to pay, a job to pay them, a house to maintain, dinner to make, a dog to walk, a car to get fixed. . . . And that's just today. Tomorrow will be more of the same, if not worse.

If you could take a walk and lie down in soft grass by

a babbling brook, it would surely help, but if you lived in a world where that were possible, you wouldn't be stressed in the first place. And if you weren't so stressed, you probably wouldn't be battling a weight problem, a weight problem that is now part of your stress.

You're on a treadmill, the kind that goes faster the faster you go just to keep up. You can't slow down enough to find the off switch. You can't slow down enough to jump off. Stress keeps flooding your system with adrenaline, pumping up your blood pressure, quickening your pulse, tensing your muscles, hiking your blood sugar— priming you for fight or flight, but since those responses are inappropriate in the twentieth century, you eat instead. You eat on the run, grabbing and gobbling whatever's handy or quick or convenient or doesn't take much thought or preparation. As a result you feel lousy, and you look like hell, and you really don't feel up to the relentlessness of this pace, but you simply don't know how to escape. You don't have the means, the physical strength, or mental commitment. One of these days, you tell yourself, you'll summon the courage to jump off. One of these days you'll take a vacation, get some much needed perspective, get healthy, make some changes.

One of these days.

Let's be realistic. Human nature being what it is, you're not going to take a flying leap off this treadmill, however taxing it is to stay on it: very, very few people make sudden, radical changes, unless external circumstances force them to. (We've seen some of our clients change their diets, their exercise habits, and their outlook literally in a matter of days, but usually because serious debilitation or even death was staring them in the eye.) What's all too likely for most people caught on the treadmill—that means you—is slow but certain degeneration, the kind of physical breakdown that sneaks up and steals your strength, your immunity, your health, your joy, and eventually your life, the kind you tend to ignore until you're too drained or diseased to reverse the process.

So we're not going to suggest you get a new life by turning into a vegetarian tonight and a jogger tomorrow. Major changes take time if they're to stick. Experience teaches us that baby steps—little, purposeful alterations in daily routine—nudge you gradually but certainly off your present self-destructive course and onto the road of permanent well-being.

And the first step? We're going to show you how to hit the off switch on the treadmill. We're going to show you how to give yourself a little hiatus, a break in the action, a restorative breather. It'll be like a mini-vacation, except you don't have to leave your everyday life to take it. We're going to help you locate that summer resort you crave, even in the dead of winter.

—YOU ARE WHAT YOU THINK—

The Feeling Light strategy is always the same: First, we help you detoxify and nourish your body so that it may heal itself. Then we help you balance and build your flow of vital energy. And then we show you how to stop sabotaging your well-being by getting you to let go of poisonous thoughts and latch onto positive, empowering ones.

People come to us not to escape their problems but to find and assert control over them. Either they're sick and have grown tired of waiting for others to heal them, or they're in pain and have grown desperate in an attempt to manage it, or they're stressed (and overweight, underweight, chronically tired, depressed, or addicted) and have run out of ways to cope or feel in control enough to cope.

Basically, we teach them how to relax. Because if a person can't calm down, they can't be in control. And a person out of control will eat or not eat until the body is so out of whack it can't fend off disease or perform as it was intended. The vicious cycle of physical maladies—weight, fatigue, and degenerative disease—can begin or end with the mind.

HOW TO RELAX

- Sit comfortably in a chair with your feet resting flat on the floor. The room should be quiet, or humming with quiet music or white noise.
- Close your eyes.
- Now, starting at the top of your head, you're going to work down your body, systematically locating and consciously letting go of tension. Focus your mind's eye on your forehead: are your brows knitted? If so, contract them as tight as you can and then release them. Consider your facial muscles: Are you grimacing? If so, screw up your features as hard as you can and let go. It may take two or three tries. Move on to your neck: Are you straining to keep your head level? If so, let your head drop to your chest, or wherever it feels most comfortable.
- Keep working down, clenching trouble spots—your hands, for instance—and releasing them. Take your time. Be thorough.
- Visualize this: You're a rag doll. You're an invertebrate. The only energy you're expending is for breathing.
- Become conscious of your breath. See it, feel it, focus on it as it comes in through your nose, expands your belly, vents back out through your nose. Concentrate

on this involuntary rhythm. Think only about your breathing.

Ah, but unbidden thoughts rush in, right? Of course they do. You're thinking of who you have to call when you get up, or errands you have to run, or people you have to confront. Trivial things. Critical things. Random thoughts. Distracting, disturbing thoughts.

No matter. You're perfectly normal. Don't expect an empty mind. Expect, instead, to have thoughts compete for your attention; just keep placing them into the out box, because you need to breathe. That's the work of the moment. That's what needs your full attention right now.

"I just keep telling myself, 'That thought will be there later,' " *says Lynn, the Feeling Light participant who's kicked drug and* *alcohol addictions and is now using stress reduction techniques* *to help her take off 100 pounds. "As soon as I catch myself* *thinking about having to call my lawyer, I focus back on feeling* *my breath, feeling my stomach move, feeling the tension just* *float away—and it does, I can literally feel my vertebrae cracking* *and my neck freeing up."*

What helps, says Lynn, is having a quiet place to go: She *uses her guest room, which she has fixed up with a tape player* *for quiet music, seashells she likes looking at, candles, and lace* *doilies. "When I'm having trouble focusing, I think, 'Why'd I* *bother to come in here if I'm going to think about all that stuff* *I came in here to escape? I may as well leave if I'm not going* *to let go of that stuff, and I've made it so nice in here, I don't* *want to leave.' "*

You don't have to have an actual room set up for this purpose. A quiet place can be your desk at work, your car, a park bench. And you don't need to banish all thoughts from your head to "succeed" at this. There's no failing at it; there's just improvement over time. Concentration is a lost art only to those who stop looking for it. You're not trying to force your mind to be quiet; you're simply searching—methodically, persistently, routinely—for the quiet that's already there. It's a matter of learning how to be present *in the moment*. It's a matter of centering your attention on the here and now.

MAINSTREAM MEDICINE?

Wait a minute, you're saying. *This is meditation!*

Yup. And it's not just for maharishis, Buddhist monks, New Age evangelists, or alternative lifestylers.

Just the act of doing it can be more physiologically restful than sleep, says David Posen, M.D., a psychiatrist whose ten tips for stress management list daily meditation second only to exercise in effectiveness. Meditation is proven effective even where stress levels are so debilitating that tranquilizers are usually prescribed. In a study conducted by Jon Kabat-Zinn, head of the Stress Reduction Center at University of Massachusetts Medical College, 20 out of 22 patients suffering from severe anxiety disorder successfully conquered anxiety, depression, panic disorders, and agoraphobia strictly through group meditation training over a three-week period.

In fact, meditation, and not medication, is the treatment recommended by the National Institutes of Health for bringing down high blood pressure. Today meditation is used in conjunction with radiation and chemotherapy to treat cancer, since a landmark study by Carl Simonton, M.D., showed better remission rates among patients who practiced daily "mindfulness"—who consistently visualized their cancer cells being overwhelmed and ultimately defeated by their own immune system.

Regular meditation has been shown even to extend life span. In a study conducted by Ellen Langer of Harvard University and Charles Alexander of Maharishi International University, octogenarians in eight Boston nursing homes who were taught to practice transcendental meditation twenty minutes a day were all still alive three years later, while 38 percent of their nonpracticing peers had died.

But perhaps the most compelling reason to try meditation is the one we've been citing all along: you need a break. The pace of your life is literally killing you, driving you to eat, not allowing you to exercise, disrupting your sleep, denying you the simple sensation of well-being that makes life worth living. There's no way you can summon inspiration, let alone act on it, when you're in the grip of this frenzy. You're moving so fast that you can't see where you're going. You're moving so fast that you can't see how to make the kind of qualitative, life-affirming changes you need in order to slow down and actually *choose* a direction. In a word, you're out of control.

Meditation can restore your sense of control. Meditation can give you the perspective you need to put everything stressing you in its proper place. Meditation can give you the kind of peace you need to resist destroying yourself with food. Our clients both in and out of Feeling Light have put it to the test, and they don't have any more time than you do.

"I deal with irrational people in a high-pressure environment all day long," explains Marilyn, 54, owner and proprietor of a children's shoe store. "I find it easier to remain calm and pleasant around them when I keep my focus on who I am, and keep in mind their relative importance in my life—they're not worth my well-being. That's what meditation is giving me: the realization that I'm not a victim, that I can take charge of my own life."

*   *   *

"Control is a big issue in my life," echoes Lynn. "When things don't go my way—if I get to an airport in Mexico and find the car rental agency we've booked with is twenty miles away—I start flipping out, not because there aren't plenty of agencies right there in the airport, but because things just didn't go according to my plan.

"Meditation, for me, is a way of regaining control so I can look at a situation more clearly. I shut my eyes, take a couple of deep breaths, and step back just enough to realize, 'This isn't as critical as your letting it get to you.' I'm learning that not everything is a federal offense."

MANTRAS AND MINDFULNESS

Back to focusing on your breath.

There's nothing magical or mystical about your breath. It's just that it happens to be intrinsic to your life, a central action that keeps you centered when you focus on it. Your breath becomes what is called a mantra: a singular word, phrase, concept, or action that through repetition keeps dragging you back to that centered place. Allow yourself anywhere from five to twenty minutes daily to focus on a mantra, and you'll clean out your mind of harmful thoughts as effectively as a fast will cleanse your body of toxic wastes (more on this later). You're going to harbor doubts about your technique: don't worry about it. Don't even practice with the expectation of results; over time, they'll become evident. Just Do It.

If sitting quietly in a quiet place makes you too self-conscious or antsy, then consider active meditation. Active meditation means simply that your mantra will be a voluntary motion rather than something involuntary like breathing, or something abstract like concentrating on a sound or word or phrase. The trick is to choose a "mindless" activity and make it "mindful," not by letting your thoughts wander to more interesting things. Instead focus on the repetitive action itself. Washing dishes can be a springboard for emptying your mind, provided you concentrate on the series of sudsing/rinsing motions required. So can taking a shower. Some people find that pushing a lawn mower up and down in rows or around and around in laps induces an almost trancelike state if they keep their mind on the mowing.

For others, walking becomes the vehicle: instead of mindlessly putting one foot in front of the other while talking, or looking at the scenery, they concentrate on their footfalls—maybe saying "left" every time their left foot hits the ground, maybe concentrating on rolling from heel to toe, maybe imagining they are walking on flowers. Exercise of any sort can lend itself to this kind of mindfulness, but certainly some are more gently repetitive than others. Tai Chi Chuan, an ancient form of circular, rhythmic movement (which we'll introduce you to it in a later chapter), is a prime example of meditation through movement.

But who has time for all this?

Building time into your life for meditation is actually quite easy if you consider how many "mindless" activities fill any given day. Just see each one of these activities as an opportunity for mindfulness. Waiting for a delayed flight to take off can mean hours wasted in an airport and a mounting case of stress . . . or it can offer the perfect meditative walk up and down the concourses. Ditto for having your hair done, or your teeth cleaned. Even eating—so often an action we barely think about, shoveling food in, boring our way through a bag of chips—offers meditative possibilities. Instead of wolfing your food, take time to register how it smells, how it looks, how it feels in your mouth. Concentrate on how your teeth move as you chew, how your throat muscles move as you swallow. (For a revelatory experience, try peeling and sectioning an orange, dwelling exclusively on its smell and texture.) At least one meal a week—one meal a day would be ideal—should be consumed "mindfully," meaning you turn off or tune out the TV, the phone, the doorbell, the mail or newspapers on the table, and all the other distractions so that you may concentrate wholly on the act of eating: on the pleasurable ritual of putting healthful food in your mouth and vital nourishment in your body.

It is the constant division and fragmentation of our attention—thinking about one thing while doing another—that undermines our ability to enjoy what each moment in time and place affords us. Life itself can be a meditation, if only we discipline ourselves to be utterly present every moment, to be *mindful* of our every thought, every word, every action.

MEDITATION AND AFFIRMATION

We use meditation in Feeling Light to help our clients refrain from eating—from eating the wrong food, from eating too much food, from eating for emotional comfort. We get them to center themselves, to seize control of their impulses, by concentrating on their breath—an effective mantra anytime, anywhere. But we also give them a list of affirmations to be studied, meditated upon, memorized, or simply repeated to the point where, whether our clients believe in them or not, they hear them at times of emotional weakness.

When, for example, the deli truck comes to her office each day, laden with pastries and bags of snack food, our client Tracy hears a little voice saying over and over, "I will put only clean and healthy food into my body"—and she resists buying the dough- nut she had her eye on. For Marilyn, who successfully rid herself of urinary tract infections and the raft of antibiotics prescribed for them, the affirmation she hears is, "I take responsibility for my physical self, my wellness, and my health." For Lynn, the mantra is very simple: "I am in control."

Affirmations are powerful statements of belief. Whether or not you believe in their power, it's important to read them out loud to yourself each day—even memorize them. The idea is to create a consciousness you may not have, a voice you most definitely need to hear. Through recitation, you will create that voice, that bee in your bonnet whose dron- ing will drown out the "I *want*" whine that drives you to eat.

Here's the list we hand out. Copy it. Post it. Commit it to memory. Recite the list out loud twice a day. Suspend dis- belief.

- With every breath I take I am healing myself.
- With every breath I am going deeper into my belly and into my blood flow.
- I am revealing a clearer, healthier, happier me.
- I am in control.
- I take responsibility for my physical self, my wellness, and my health.
- I eat to nourish my mind, body, and spirit.
- I put only good, healthy, clean food into this vehicle that carries me through life knowing that this is the only physical vehicle that I have.
- I take care to keep it lean, responsive, and strong, so I may glide effortlessly through my life to feel peaceful and well.

• I am learning to love and nurture my body, and with every deep breath that I take, I am healing.

Feel free to modify these or add your own. The most important thing is to hear or see these affirmations in a weak moment—as you're opening the refrigerator, or passing that vending machine. They'll help strengthen your willpower to fight a craving and thus keep you on the path to wellness.

DOING IT WRONG

You can't.

There isn't, as we've already noted, a "right" way to meditate. Having a slew of random thoughts skitter across your mind while trying to clear a space there is absolutely typical. With practice, you get better at banishing them. With practice, there's more peace in your session than distraction.

Don't obsess about "rules," either: you don't have to keep your eyes shut, you don't have to be in a quiet room, you don't have to think of this relaxation technique as meditation, and you don't have to focus on your breath. For some, looking at ocean waves and hearing them crash, or watching leaves shimmer in the wind, or staring at clouds offers an ideal opportunity for meditation. Others do best when listening to the voice of another person, either in a meditative class or on a tape. There aren't "better" kinds of meditation; there is only what works for you, in your particular circumstances.

Above all, don't let meditation's mystical associations spook you. Meditation in our program is simply a tool in the toolbox, a means of getting you to that balanced place where life has meaning, joy, and peace. It's one of several tools to get you through, say, that three o'clock slump in the workday; to calm a tortuous craving for chocolate; and to enhance the quality and quantity of your days here on this planet.

And it's perhaps the best tool we know of to silence that inner naysayer, that voice that undermines your every attempt to change. You can change. You can bring your eating and your life back under control.

It's mind over matter.

CHAPTER THREE

Readying the Body

Stand, Breathe, Stretch, Move!

Stand up and take a deep breath.

Really deep.

Exhale. Slowly.

Now look at your feet. Feel how you're standing. Are you favoring one foot over another? Is your weight shifted so as to push out one hip?

Let's start over. Stand on *two* feet, this time. Make sure you're distributing your weight perfectly, so that each foot is getting exactly the same load. Don't rock back on your heels, or forward on the balls of your feet. Try and feel rooted to the earth through every cell in your soles. Drop your shoulders. Relax your hands. Hold your head as if it were suspended from the ceiling by a thread anchored to the very crown of your skull.

Now focus on how this feels.

You should feel balanced. Centered. Without strain, any-where. Doesn't this feel good?

Count on feeling even better as we progress, because this whole book is about balance—balanced weight, balanced nutrition, emotional composure, and physiological equilib-rium. Right now you're doing a small thing—just standing on two feet. But like many of the changes we're going to propose, it's a small action with huge ramifications: you're no longer out of alignment, throwing your weight un-evenly, throwing your spine off line, stressing ligaments, tendons, cartilage, and joints, or blocking circulation. Your organs are getting the food and nourishment they need to perform optimally, so you'll feel more energy. There's no strain on anything, so you'll feel no pain.

Now focus on your breathing. How you breathe is an-other "little" thing you can adjust ever so slightly to reap tremendous benefits. We're going to prepare you for bet-ter, more oxygenating breathing by strengthening your di-aphragm. That's the muscle singers develop so they can belt out entire arias to thousands of people in an amphi-theater without the aid of a microphone. Your diaphragm resides above your belly, below your breastbone. You're going to exercise it by doing something we call "bellows breathing." You're going to inhale and exhale as though you were blowing on a fire, using your diaphragm as the bellows.

First, place your hands across your torso, palms over the lower part of your rib cage, fingertips meeting just below your sternum. That's the diaphragm. Feel how it moves as you breathe. Now, using this muscle alone to fill your lungs, breathe in and out rapidly, almost as though you were panting. Relax everything else. Your shoulders shouldn't be going up and down, and your chest shouldn't be expanding much. Allow your diaphragm to draw quick, shallow breaths for thirty seconds or more, up to a minute or so. (Stop if you feel dizzy.)

Do this once or twice a day, ideally upon waking (it'll give you an oxygen rush) or at the beginning of your exercise routine, or at the onset of that late-afternoon slump (you'll wake up your brain). It's also good for clearing headaches. In a week or so, you'll have toned your diaphragm so that each breath you take is bigger, better, and more oxygenating—and you won't even be conscious of it, just as you're not conscious now of how shallowly you normally breathe. Small investment, big payoff.

STRETCHING

You barely have the time to exercise, let alone stretch. Or so you think.

We're not talking about an hour of yoga. We're as busy as you are, and just as reluctant to carve out a chunk of time spent on the floor. So here's what we do, for a minute in the morning, a minute in the evening, or a minute at our desks: we aerate our spines.

By that we mean we allow the spaces between our vertebrae to "breathe," so that blood can flow and nourish the critical tissues and nerve pathways of our spine. Start by standing squarely on two feet, as we've discussed. Gradually drop your chin to your chest, relying solely on gravity to pull on your head. Your head should feel like a bowling ball, an eight- or ten-pound free weight. Let that weight pull your head further down: first your neck will yield, then vertebra by vertebra, your spine will curve. Allow your arms to fall away from your sides. Give in to the bowling ball until you've reached the extent of your flexibility; that may mean your hands are two feet off the floor, or resting on the carpet. Hang there, anchored by your feet and heavy head.

Bend your knees slightly and exhale. As you start to inhale, straighten your knees. Bend and exhale; inhale and straighten. Do this about five times. Breathe slowly.

Your head should still be hanging as though it were way too heavy for your rag doll body to lift. But now you're going to lever it up, one vertebra at a time. Starting at the base of your spine, begin to rise by stacking up your vertebrae. You want to pile one vertebra on top of another as if each were a block and you were building a tower of blocks. Picture this tower in your mind as you build it. When you run out of blocks, place your head carefully on top.

You should feel that good, centered sensation of balance again. Your back and neck have just had a mini-massage, where bloodflow is restored and nerve pathways are freed from skeleto-muscular constriction.

And guess what? This whole stretch has taken a minute. No more than five, certainly. You're energized. You've gotten a quick fix. Maybe you've stifled a craving that would otherwise have forced you to raid the kitchen cupboards. Most importantly, you've restored mobility to a site where all too many people lack it, mostly from disuse. Think about how your knee would feel if you locked it in a cast for an hour, let alone a day, a week, or months at a stretch. Either it'd be mighty stiff or utterly incapable of movement. That's how most people treat their spines, without even realizing it. And when your spine locks up . . . well, you know *exactly* what we're talking about.

DRY BRUSHING

Your skin is not just a protective hide that keeps blood in and germs out. It's the largest organ of the human body, the one that encases all the others. You can't see through it to gauge internal health, but you don't need to: it mirrors what's going on inside. Of course, some skin aberrations— wrinkles, freckles, moles, age spots, varicose veins, spider veins—can be attributed to too much sun, childbearing, heredity, and daily wear and tear.

But a lot of what we see and lament is actually toxic waste surfacing—what dermatologists call "nonspecific dermatitis." Your skin is largely an organ of elimination, whereby toxins picked up from tissues and circulated by the blood and lymph are deposited in the epithelial layers if they're not filtered out by the liver and kidneys. If, in turn, those epithelial layers don't get shed and regener- ated, the toxins just sit ·there. Pretty soon, you've got buildup. Over time, you've got degradation of skin tone and elasticity. Or worse: the toxins get reabsorbed into your system, along with new ones contributed by pollution and solar radiation.

Toxicity, as we'll discuss, can be a major impediment to weight management. In subsequent chapters, we'll be shar- ing with you many different ways to purge these toxins— through fasting, through herbs, and through nutritional supplements—but there's an immediate, mechanical way to start the cleansing process, and it's called dry brushing.

Buy a loofah—those natural sponges people often use as exfoliating washcloths—and use it dry. (We don't recommend plastic brushes or plastic sponges.) You're going to scrub your skin every day, before you get in the shower. Brush in one direction only; stroke your skin so that you're always stroking *toward* your heart. That is, wrists to elbows, elbows to shoulder, neck to shoulders, ankles to knees, knees to thighs, abdomen to chest. You're accomplishing several things with this "dry brushing": an exfoliation of dead epithelial cells, along with their toxic load; a stimulation of circulation, both blood and lymph; and a gentle stretching. Overall, it's like a massage.

—BODYWORKS—

Speaking of which, treat yourself to a decent bodywork session by a qualified therapist, or do self massage (see Appendix). If nothing else, it will awaken you to your own body, to sensations that abuse and disuse may have dulled or blotted out. Body readiness is in part body awareness. You know what you look like, of course—but are you conscious of how you feel when you move? When you sit? When you relax—or fail to relax?

Massage restores circulation, which in some cases can mean relief from muscular knotting or pain. For those in pain, massage can be the means of escaping the vicious cycle: you're in pain so you don't move, and because you don't move, blood doesn't circulate into the ailing area, so you can't heal, and you don't get any pain relief.

We endorse whatever kind of bodywork you enjoy or find gives you relief. In fact, we suggest you experiment with different methods, to find one that works for you. Different techniques are suited to different people; we firmly believe this. A partial list of options would include:

- Swedish massage
- Shiatsu
- Reflexology
- Feldenkrais method
- Deep-tissue massage
- Craniosacral therapy
- Trager method
- Alexander technique
- Aston patterning
- Reiki
- Rolfing
- Acupressure
- Chiropractic
- Yoga therapy
- Jin Shin Do
- Rubenfeld Synergy
- Myofascial Relief

We're also keen on sauna, if you've got access to one. A sauna or steam bath can optimize the effects of dry brushing and massage. Hot steam speeds the toxic removal process by stimulating circulation and causing you to perspire. Heat opens your pores so that you literally sweat out the poisons. It's also relaxing. However, high temperatures are not beneficial to everyone—pregnant women, children, and those with heart conditions should take a pass on saunas and steam baths.

EXERCISE

If you thought we were going to tell you that you don't need any, you're living in a dream world.

On the other hand, if we thought we could convince you to go buy a NordicTrack and spend an hour on it each day, then *we're* living in a dream world. (Congratulations if you're actually skiing on one. Most people we know use their bikes or tracks as an extra place to hang clothes.)

For those of you who are exercising regularly, keep up

the good work. But for those of you who aren't, keep this in mind: a little bit of exercise is better than none at all. Daily exercise *of some sort* is vital to life, not just to weight management. We're not talking anything strenuous or grueling. We don't subscribe to the "no pain, no gain" fitness mantra. We know all too well that if exercise is torturous, you're not going to keep at it. In fact, if exercise doesn't have some pleasant component, some immediate reward, some aspect of feeling good, we know you won't even bother.

Later in this book we're going to introduce you to *Tai Chi Chuan*, a gentle system of movements anybody of any age can do every day for the rest of his or her life. It's precisely the kind of "exercise" we'd like to turn you on to, because you'll reap so many rewards from what appears to be very little exertion. But in the event you're not ready to learn something new, or you're feeling at all reluctant, there are, of course, other options.

REBOUNDING

Rebounding is simply jumping up and down. For forty dollars, you can get a mini-trampoline at any sporting goods store and bounce your way to better health. You don't have to be an athlete, or even very coordinated. Gentle jumping at first is best; when your stamina and coordination improve, you can jump with more vigor, or add one- or three-pound handweights to your routine. Move your arms back and forth, swing them in opposite directions, bring them over your head, do bicep or tricep curls, or any variation you enjoy. Rebounding with light handweights is one of our favorite workouts, improving aerobic capacity, upper body strength, and overall muscle tone.

Because it hikes your metabolism, it's a real pound-shedder. Five minutes a day is a good start; if you like it, build up to a twenty- or thirty-minute workout. Listen to music, watch TV, or take your trampoline outside. When you get off the rebounder, keep moving or walking until your heart slows down to a normal pace.

WALKING

Here's the beauty of that daily constitutional: everyone knows how to do it. Everyone can afford it. Everyone can benefit from it. No equipment required, unless you count shoes. Whether you go around the block, around a track, or around town, you're getting your blood moving, nourishing your every cell with oxygen and with the food you'd otherwise store as fat. It's so unstrenuous you can talk at the same time, which means you can enjoy walking as a social opportunity as well as a health tonic.

Don't have time for a twenty-minute walk? Then break it up into three- and five-minute bursts, the kind of mini-walk we'd all be doing now if we weren't such a car dependent, sedentary people. You'd be surprised how much walking you *don't* do. If you're like most Americans, you'll circle a parking lot, looking for a spot closest to the door of the store you intend to enter. Or you'll take an elevator, even if your destination is a floor or two away. Or you'll opt for drive-through service to spare you the few steps from car to cash register. You'll get in the car to pick up milk even if the market is four blocks away.

Look at it this way: If you take the car because you "don't have time," consider the time you've spent and will spend dieting; the time you spend at a doctor's office to figure out why you feel lousy and have no energy; the time you spend at an expensive fat farm or fitness club; and the time you're shaving off your life span. Walking is a fundamental maintenance measure, a minimal investment in quality of life, if not quantity. Use it or lose it.

If you're already walking, step up the pace for more aerobic benefit. Better yet, get yourself some of those one- or two-pound handweights and swing your arms as you stride for a whole-body workout. Women, in particular, can benefit from weight-bearing exercise, since it helps stall or prevent the onset of osteoporosis, a disease affecting millions of postmenopausal women whose bone density has deteriorated to the point of frailty. Bench-pressing is not necessary; repetitive use of one- or two-pound handweights will help keep your bones from degenerating (along with a change in diet, which we'll discuss later).

Walk, rebound, bicycle, whatever. Get moving, however slowly, however unsurely; no one is clocking you for the Olympic trials. Breathlessness is to be expected. Build up gradually; stamina will improve. Exercise regularly; if not every day, at least three times a week. A little every day is far better than a lot on weekends only, or none at all, for that matter.

Exercise is what eating is intended to fuel, once bodily functions have been seen to. If you exercise more, you'll rev up your metabolism, burning what you ingest more efficiently and using up fat stores more effectively. You'll also increase your circulation, speeding nutrients and oxygen to your cells, tissues, and organs, speeding toxins out of your body via blood and lymph. Better circulation means more energy. More energy means you feel better enough, strong enough, committed enough, to making permanent changes in what you eat, how you move, the way you live. Each little change makes the next little change that much easier, until you've effected a total mind/body transformation.

That's how real, lasting change comes about. "A thousand miles' journey," goes the popular Chinese saying, "begins from the spot under one's feet."

PART TWO

Get Set . . .

CHAPTER FOUR

Foods That Harm

The Link Between Wellness and Weight Management

In the course of our experiences, we've seen some pretty sick people. Some are literally at death's door. They come to us not necessarily because they believe in alternative therapies but because they've tried everything else and nothing is stopping or even slowing their decline. Rosario, 68, afflicted with a bone marrow disorder, was told by his hematologist that if he didn't get a transfusion and raise his red corpuscle count, he was going to die. But he was also told by his kidney doctor that if he got a transfusion, it would overload his one poorly functioning kidney and he'd die from kidney failure. "I had nowhere else to turn," he admitted to us, "and nothing to lose."

Others come not because they are dying but because they've got a malady that denies them quality of life. Mary Lynn, a 43-year-old school counselor who recently divorced her alcoholic husband of eighteen years, couldn't face getting out of bed each morning without a double dosage of antidepressants. Anne-Marie, a 34-year-old chemical engineer, was so incapacitated by vertigo from chronic ear infections that she was afraid to drive, afraid to travel, and afraid she'd never be free of the nausea and confusion that accompanied her dizziness.

These were people clearly out of whack, people who themselves wouldn't hesitate to concede that some fundamental equilibrium had gone awry. Because we believe the body heals itself, given the right working materials, we routinely address imbalance—whatever its physical manifestation—through diet. So invariably, we would ask about our clients' eating habits. And invariably, they'd get a little defensive. Most everyone insisted they ate a "balanced" diet. What, exactly, did that mean? we persisted. Well, three square meals a day, was the response. Pretty much your standard American fare.

—THE ENERGY OF FOOD—

Balance, to our way of thinking, is a state of harmony. Not a static condition, but an even and constant exchange of energy. Balance is when everything works as it should, when no one force gets out of control, when no single influence prevails. When we apply our image of balance to the human body, we see it in dynamic equilibrium: ceaselessly changing, but perfectly efficient in its continual processing of energies.

When we apply the concept of balance to diet, we see a continuum of foods, with the most healthful range in the middle and the most objectionable at the extreme ends. In our experience, and according to a 4,000-year-old Eastern tradition, people who eat foods that fall more or less dead center on this gradient tend to be physically healthy, emotionally even-tempered, and mentally balanced. Those eating foods that fall on either side of center can be healthy, provided they strive for symmetry. Those who routinely eat at the extremes rarely attain balance, let alone maintain it, and manifest, sooner or later, acute or chronic symptoms of that imbalance.

The Chinese illustrate balance with the *yin-yang* symbol, a circular swirl of opposing and attracting energies that represent the dynamic forces within Nature. This symbol, when applied to diet, classifies food according to its *yin* or *yang* qualities. Yang foods are those characterized by heat and dryness; yin foods, in contrast, are those which are cool and moist. The more yang or the more yin a food—the hotter and drier, or the colder and wetter—the further out from the neutral center the food falls. Hot or cooked foods are more yang than cold or raw foods.

In the middle—neither yin nor yang—is brown rice, thought by the Chinese to be nutritionally ideal. On either side of brown rice, comprising the middle of the gradient, are whole grains, beans, vegetables, and sea vegetables. At the yin and yang extremes, interestingly enough, are foods the scientific community has finally acknowledged to be unhealthy except in very small amounts: fats, refined sugars, alcohol, salt, and preservatives, to name a few.

There are other areas where Western science has recently validated what the Chinese have known and practiced for millennia. For example, normal human pH is ever

Most Yin	Derivatives	Dairy	Fruits and Vegetables	Light Grains	Brown Rice	Heavier Grains	Nuts & Legumes	Fish & Fowl	Meats & Eggs	Most Yang
		Cooling / alkalizing			Neutral		Warming / acidifying			

so slightly alkaline, falling at 7.3 on a scale of 1 to 14, with 1 being acid and 14, base. Those who are sick or diseased, however, have been shown to have an altered pH—blood that's too acidic, usually. Foods high in protein, such as meat, move bodily pH toward the excessively acid, while foods high in calcium (dairy products, for example) make the body more alkaline. A diet balancing food's natural acidity and alkalinity thus helps maintain health by keeping pH at its optimal, neutral level. The Chinese classification of foods as yang, yin, or neutral demonstrates an uncanny awareness of biochemistry: meat falls at the extremely yang end of the spectrum, along with other acidifying foods like fish and nuts, while dairy is perceived at the extremely yin pole, along with alkalizing foods like coffee and lemon juice (acidic in your stomach, but alkalizing on your blood pH).

Whereas Westerners rely on biochemical analysis to figure out which foods comprise good nutrition, the Chinese balance their diet by balancing the *energies* of the foods they ingest. A calorie, after all, is nothing but a measurement of heat, or energy. The calories we eat translate into the calories we "burn" in order to fuel an action. We need food in order to harness its energy to perform any action, whether it's drawing a breath or running a marathon. Food energy is thus ultimately transformed into kinetic energy, or motion. What the Chinese recognized 4,000 years ago is that energy may take many guises, but it is still energy, and it is never lost—only moved. That's why a balance of food energies brings about a balance of life forces within the human body. Since this energy, or *chi*, courses through all organic, living matter on the earth, we are, quite literally, what we eat.

And what most Americans are eating is S.A.D.—the Standard American Diet, that is.

OVERFED AND UNDERNOURISHED

Remember the four food groups?

Sure you do, unless you were born yesterday, when the Food and Drug Administration reshuffled the four-square into a pyramid. For most of this century, "balanced" meals described those which represented all four groups: meat (picture the hunk of steak), dairy (milk, eggs, butter, and ice cream), fruits and vegetables (Libby's and Green Giant, right?), and grains (anything processed in Battle Creek, Michigan).

Eat three square meals a day and drink your milk for strong muscles, bones, and teeth! The message was inescapable. We learned it at school, practiced it in the cafeteria, absorbed it from television ("a public service message"), and grew up to rear our own children on its wisdom. To this day, we believe in the four food groups' sacred premise: we *need* all that protein and calcium, because without it, our muscles will wither, our brains will starve, and our bones will wind up as delicate as doilies.

Did we never question who published and distributed all those nutritional pamphlets and workbooks we carefully crayoned at school? Did we never notice who brought us all those public service messages on TV? Did we never correlate the economic clout of the dairy and beef industries in this country with the tenacity they've shown in remaining staples of the American diet, despite overwhelming consensus that meat, milk, and eggs are our main sources of fat, calories, and cholesterol?

If the tobacco industry and its powerful lobby were to print up and hand out materials that propagandized the health benefits of smoking, we'd be up in arms. As it is, when we read that Philip Morris proclaims there is no link between smoking and lung cancer, we can barely contain ourselves: The conflict of interest is outrageous.

But when it comes to dairy products, milk and eggs define our very notion of wholesomeness. And beef—well, "It's What's For Dinner," regardless of how pumped full of hormones, saturated with antibiotics, riddled with tumors, or tainted with Mad Cow disease it may be. Beef is a First World privilege, the dietary component that separates robust Americans from starving Indians. Only in the United States would an ad campaign like "Where's the beef?" become a countrywide hue and cry. Look at our media, at the images we cherish. Cattle and dairy farmers are national icons, whether we find them on a Marlboro billboard or in a Norman Rockwell painting.

To put it mildly, the beef and dairy interests in this country have been phenomenally successful in hooking us on the merits of their products, to the point of blinding us to their health hazards. Today, 78 million Americans—20 million of them children—are at least 20 percent over their ideal weight. Fully a third of the population is at risk for developing such weight-related diseases as diabetes, colorectal and breast cancer, hypertension, stroke, and atherosclerosis—the five most lethal diseases in the United States. After smoking, excessive weight is the number one killer in America, taking 300,000 lives annually.

The federal government would have to be blind, deaf, and dumb—or heavily vested in beef and dairy interests—not to notice the correlation between our eating habits and our dying habits. George McGovern's Select Committee on Nutrition and Human Needs did report, in 1977, that "over-consumption of fat, generally, and saturated fat in particular, as well as cholesterol, sugar, salt and alcohol have been related to six of the ten leading causes of death," but the dietary goals set forth by the committee—reducing fat to 30 percent, and raising complex carbohydrate consumption to 50 percent—were deemed "controversial" and never surfaced beyond the U.S. Senate floor. Not until 1988 did Surgeon General C. Everett Koop formally and publically acknowledge the obvious. His report on nutrition and health declared *a conclusive link* between diet and the five leading causes of death and disability in the United States. Its nutritional recommendations: a diet lower in fats, sugars, and calories, and higher in complex carbohydrates, fruits, and vegetables.

We couldn't agree more.

Yet look how the Food and Drug Administration has embraced these recent recommendations. As if to undermine its own Food Guide advice—that Americans should avoid saturated fats *by avoiding the foods that contain them*— the FDA approved olestra, the indigestible fat substitute, giving manufacturer Procter & Gamble the green light to flood the supermarket shelves with nutritionally void, calorically high, "fat-free" snacks. Foods containing olestra (labeled as Olean) will be "fortified," but don't be fooled: nutrients have been added because olestra tends to strip vitamins and minerals from the gastrointestinal tract in passage. Worse, clinical trials have shown that the fake fat provokes nausea, diarrhea, cramping, and foul-smelling stools. That's because it cannot be digested by the bacteria colonizing our intestines—or any other bacteria, for that matter. The fact that olestra is nonbiodegradeable has environmentalists pointing to an imminent waste processing crisis: excreted olestra will coat water supplies like an oil slick, suffocating fish and wildlife like spilled crude. Except, crude oil eventually breaks down. Olestra does not.

Apparently our addiction to junk foods is so great that

we would sooner pollute our waterways and ravage our intestinal tracts than change our eating habits. We can't quit the fat, no matter how many foods in our cupboards proclaim themselves nonfat or low-fat. The American diet remains woefully saturated with saturated fats—those which are solid at room temperature.

- They're fats we get from animal meat and dairy products, from fast food franchises and our own frying pans.
- They lurk in our processed foods, in the form of tropical oils—coconut, palm, and palm kernel.
- They're baked into breads and then slathered on as spreads in the form of "hydrogenated" or "partially hydrogenated" oils—polyunsaturates or monounsaturates transformed by high heat into more stable, more durable, *saturated* solids such as vegetable shortening or margarine.

Americans who switched to margarine in an attempt to cut back on butter's evils unwittingly introduced something much worse: trans-fatty acids, substances created by hydrogenization, which are thought to block our uptake of essential fatty acids, which are just that—essential to health.

The terrible irony is that in our attempts to get rid of the fat that's bad we inadvertently wind up getting rid of the few fats that are good. Essential fatty acids (EFAs)— linoleic and linolenic acid, for example—are literally the building blocks of life. Cells cannot be constructed without them. An EFA deficiency, as we will discuss in our chapter on foods that heal, is thought to be one of the prime reasons why many of us overeat in the first place.

And we do overeat. Forget the "fat gene," "carbohydrate sensitivity," "insulin resistance," and all the other excuses we've dreamed up to account for our condition. Americans are fat—and growing fatter—because we eat the wrong foods and too much of them. Today, 1 in 3 adults is overweight, up from 1 in 4 in 1980; 1 in 5 teens is obese. In 1993, former surgeon general Dr. Koop, alarmed by the 100 billion dollars that the obesity "epidemic" costs the United States annually in health care and lost productivity, spearheaded Shape Up America, a campaign whose goal was to make healthy weight a national priority. The campaign is based on the notion that if only Americans understood how *dangerous* excess weight is— instead of how unbecoming—they would suddenly throw out their remote controls, eat sensibly, use the stairs instead of the elevator, and shed those extra pounds.

In other words, says the former surgeon general, if you lose the weight and keep it off, you'll be a lot healthier and a lot less likely to die of obesity-related diseases.

So what's wrong with this thinking? Ask Mary, 50, a participant in our weekly Feeling Light workshops. Mary signed up for the program's promise of better health: she suffered from irritable bowel syndrome (IBS), high cholesterol, and high blood pressure. In the course of the program, she got rid of the IBS, lowered her cholesterol count, and reduced her hypertension to the point of going off her medication. And in the course of getting well, she lost thirty pounds.

"We're taught to think that if we could only lose the weight, we'd be healthy," notes Mary, who yo-yoed for years as a Lean Line member. "Feeling Light's convinced me that just the opposite is true: If you get healthy, you'll lose the weight."

BALANCE AND WELLNESS

We can't stress this enough: if you're plagued with illness or unable to manage your weight, then you are manifesting imbalance. Getting well—or losing weight—is a matter of recalibrating your body's fundamental equilibrium. To do that you've got to minimize the sabotaging effects of mental and emotional stress and maximize the healing effects of biochemical change. That means detoxifying and then nourishing the body with specific foods and supplements; boosting immunity with herbs to combat infection; tempering emotional excess with calming flower essences, meditative exercises, and breathing exercises; and opening up the energy pathways of the body with acupuncture, self acupressure, or tai chi to free it of pain and unhealthy cravings and to facilitate circulation of healing nutrients and oxygen.

The more you heal, the better you feel. The better you feel, the more likely you are to treat your whole self with respect and care. The more balanced your diet—according to the guidelines we've established—the less you will crave harmful foods, and the easier it will be to balance your weight and keep it moderate. Achieving equilibrium of mind and body is like balancing an old-fashioned set of scales: both ends wind up in the air, buoyant and seemingly weightless.

That's the Feeling Light philosophy in a nutshell. Wellness leads to weight management. Not the other way around.

A TRULY BALANCED DIET

Now let's discuss dietary guidelines. The FDA Food Guide Pyramid is not so much wrong as it is a compromise: if you follow its recommendations on servings of complex carbohydrates and fruits and vegetables, you'll also be pretty much eating within the central range of the yin-yang gradient we've described. Both sets of dietary guidelines find whole grains preferable to rolled, cracked, or bleached grains, because all the nutrients and fiber remain intact. Both sets of dietary guidelines also warn against the perils of refined sugar, which has been stripped of its fiber and nutrients. For a fact, foods eaten in their whole, original form are more satisfying—because they're bulkier, and because their nutritional complement answers our cravings at their deepest level. What makes us insatiable are the denatured, processed, *white* foods—white flour, white sugar, white table salt, white fat (like Crisco). Those foods, nutritionally barren as they are, rekindle our enthusiasm for . . .

Meat and dairy. These groups occupy the third tier of the Food Pyramid, and the outer ranges on the yin-yang gradient. But whereas the FDA recommends that you switch from whole milk to 1 percent or skim, and from ice cream to fat-free frozen yogurt, and from cheese to a low-fat version, we're saying work toward eliminating the category altogether, except as a condiment (a little milk in your tea, a little Parmesan on your pasta, etc.). And whereas the FDA urges you to substitute turkey for bacon and bologna, we're urging you to move toward an almost meatless diet: no more than three animal-protein meals per week.

Note that we say, "move toward." Few carnivores become vegetarians, or even almost-vegetarians, overnight—and we're not telling you to. Some people are not meant to be vegetarians. Some individuals most certainly can benefit from meat's expansive properties. We're suggesting you cut back, without obsessing about absolutes; Feeling

Light is about moderation, meaning some meat and dairy can figure in your diet. But let's be clear on what we mean by meat, and what we mean by "cutting back." Beef, lamb, chicken, pork, veal, turkey, and fish are all sources of animal protein—that is, meat. We're suggesting that only three meals per week—3 out of every 21 meals, that is—include animal protein. Americans are very conscious of the perils of eating too much red meat, but we want to raise that consciousness: chicken is meat! so is fish! (Take a look at our weekly menus in the Epilogue.)

Experience has shown us that wellness and weight management are maximally achieved by a diet of grains, pastas, fruits, and vegetables, but how much and how fast you move toward this not-very-meaty middle is entirely up to you. What we have observed, however, is that the more extreme your imbalance, in terms of weight or illness, the more dramatic the rate of your healing process if you cut out the meat and dairy.

> *Consider Rosario, the gentleman we mentioned who was disabled by a bone marrow disease and a failing kidney. Rosario, a confirmed meat-and-potatoes man for sixty-eight years, followed our advice and went cold turkey to a diet of vegetables and brown rice. He had more incentive than most: he was so debilitated that he couldn't stand up. Rosario also consented to acupuncture treatments—something, he says, "I never would have pursued if I hadn't reached rock bottom."*
>
> *Within two days of the acupuncture, he felt markedly better. Within two weeks of going off all meat and dairy, says Rosario, "I felt better than I had in six months," and he went back to work. His red corpuscle count rose. His doctors couldn't believe it.*
>
> *"People at work have asked me, what have I been*

doing that I'm so much more energetic, so much more alive," says Rosario. "I tell them it's a combination of nutrition and acupuncture.

"Now, I'd be lying if I said I didn't miss my steak and my wife's good cooking," he adds. "But I don't think I'll ever go back. If I hadn't made those changes, I don't think I'd be talking to you today."

This is no voodoo magic. Going off meat gave Rosario more energy, we suspect, by relieving the load on his one poor kidney. The body breaks down protein into amino acids, which are then absorbed into the bloodstream. These nutrients alter blood pH from its slightly alkaline state to one of such acidity that the bones are prompted to release their stores of calcium, a natural buffer, as a means of restoring tolerable pH. That calcium, once it's done its job in the blood, must then be filtered out by the kidneys and excreted in urine. In some cases, the amounts of calcium and uric acid thrown off by the kidneys is so excessive that stones form—a destructive and painful condition afflicting almost exclusively those who eat a lot of meat. Ditto for gout, a disease interestingly on the rise among women, as well as men. Study after study confirms that protein adversely affects kidney tissue and function. Little wonder, then, that Rosario was on the brink of dialysis.

Meat does contribute iron to our systems, which is probably why we associate it with strength and robust blood. In fact, for some of our critically deficient clients, meat is something we actually urge them to eat. But for the vast majority of us, animal flesh is so difficult to digest that our bodies wind up with an energy deficit rather than surplus. And in Rosario's case, he literally couldn't afford the energies needed to digest and process all that protein.

—HOW MUCH IS TOO MUCH?—

Well, consider the well-ingrained four-food-group "ideal" of incorporating protein at every meal. A meal in America just doesn't seem "complete" without meat and/or dairy. Milk and eggs at breakfast, milk and tuna for lunch, milk and steak and ice cream for dinner—it all adds up to a whopping 30 percent (frequently more) of our daily caloric intake. The FDA is currently suggesting we halve that, to 15 percent, or two to three servings a day instead of six. The World Health Organization, garnering statistics on protein consumption and diet-related disease worldwide, reports that protein should account for only 5 *percent* of our daily intake. If that percentage sounds too low to support adequate brain function, consider this: the protein content of human breastmilk, which meets the nutritional needs of an infant during its most critical growth and development period, is 5 percent.

If you're still not convinced, consider that the United States leads the world in protein consumption—and in the incidence of cancer, specifically cancer of the colon, breast, pancreas, and prostate. The longest-lived cultures in the world are, ironically, Third World peoples such as those who live in the Andes of Ecuador, in the Himalayas of Pakistan, and along the Black Sea in Russia. These populations, despite the harshness of their environments, thrive well past the age of eighty. And what they have in common is a vegetarian or almost meatless diet, with protein consumption at *less than 2 percent*.

Another clue may be found in our teeth, twenty-eight of which are designed for grinding grains or cutting veg-

etable matter. Only four teeth, the canines, a
to tearing animal flesh. Purely carnivorous
as dogs and cats have not only the teeth for such a diet
but also the bowels. Unlike our twisting, twining, pocket-
filled intestines, which are some six times our body length,
those of, say, a lion, are more like stovepipe—short,
smooth, straight, and engineered to speed food matter
along its way without the aid of fiber. Our intestinal tract
is perfect for extracting nutrients from plant matter, because all those nooks and crannies allow cellulose-rich
foods to linger long enough to be broken down. But those
same nooks and crannies allow meat to putrefy, because
in the absence of fiber, meat doesn't move along. Putre-
fying food attracts unhealthy bacteria—interlopers which
crowd out the resident bacteria responsible for good digestion. And those unhealthy bacteria, while feeding,
throw off carcinogenic waste products. Both the absence
of "good" bacteria and the concentration of toxic waste is
thought to cause colon cancer in meat eaters; in contrast,
colon cancer is unknown among Seventh Day Adventists,
who follow a high-carb, high-fiber, vegetarian diet from
birth.

THE PROTEIN DIET

Human beings derive everything they need from three
sources: carbohydrates, proteins, and fats. A balanced diet
draws from each of these macronutrients, although not in
equal proportion. The optimal ratio of complex carbohydrates and plant matter to protein and fat should be about
7 to 1. In terms of preventing disease and maximizing
health, we believe the facts speak overwhelmingly in favor
of such a ratio.

But what about weight loss? For much of the past decade, the emphasis in dieting has been persistently anti-

carbohydrate. The notion that someone can be "allergic" to carbohydrates, or "sensitive" to them is a more recent variation on this same theme. The enduring popularity of the protein diet may well lie in the fact that people don't have to alter their habits much: cutting out fruits, starchy vegetables, bread, and pasta in favor of steak and cheese has proved remarkably easy for the typical dieter. Then there's the fact that weight loss can be immediate and dramatic, largely because protein leaches the water retained in tissues.

But this diet is also the one likeliest to backfire. For one thing, along with the water that protein pulls from bodily tissue, come trace minerals called electrolytes, without which you literally cannot move a muscle, along with calcium and potassium, which are also critical players in the ionic exchange necessary for muscle contraction. The ensuing weakness, shakiness, "burning" sensation, and desperate lassitude drives many a protein dieter to binge on foods high in fat and simple carbohydrates, thereby undoing the weight loss and further skewing biochemical balance.

Severe constipation is one of the first signs of this imbalance: animal sources of protein utterly lack fiber, which is universally understood to be critical in maintaining bowel health and warding off cancer of the colon, among other diseases. Those wishing to lose weight should realize that you can't feel light if you can't move your bowels without violent chemical laxatives.

If by some remarkable discipline or emotional disorder the dieter succeeds in staying on the all-protein regimen, the effects can be life-threatening. Ask Rebecca, 24, whose all-protein diet "just went way out of control." She cut out all carbohydrates and fats ("it was the latest thing") and subsisted on cottage cheese, tuna, and egg whites for six months. "Some afternoons, I couldn't get out of my chair," she recalls. "I'd go to bed with this burning, starving feeling every night." Finally, she says, "I got to the point where physically and emotionally, every part of me shut down."

To this day, the effects of that diet haunt her. She's being treated with acupuncture to relieve chronic bloating and stomach distress. There's no telling how her kidneys and liver have held up to months of strain from filtering out vital minerals and the by-products of burned body tissue; Rebecca may well have suffered ketosis, a highly toxic condition that leaves the kidneys permanently damaged from processing waste products that were never intended to be waste. And her diet may well have selected her as a candidate for osteoporosis: her bone calcium stores were bound to have been ransacked by the relentless onslaught of acid-forming foods.

CALCIUM AND OSTEOPOROSIS

Okay, so maybe you'll commit to cutting back on your meat quotient. But speaking of osteoporosis—do you dare cut out dairy?

Chances are pretty good that you've made a conscious effort to *increase* your dairy consumption these days, at least if you're female. If you're lactose intolerant—as many people are—you probably take pills with the enzyme lactase to alleviate the gas, bloating, and diarrhea that milk products give you, rather than just avoid dairy products because you don't want to lose out on all that calcium. Calcium is what contributes to bone density. Without sufficient calcium, you've been told, your bones will deteriorate with age until your spine collapses and your hips snap like twigs in the act of getting out of bed. What with the prevalence of osteoporosis among postmenopausal women in this country, you're not about to eliminate dairy, no matter how much discomfort it causes.

In *Diet for a New America*, author John Robbins debunks the osteoporosis-calcium argument by noting that native Eskimo women, whose fish and fishbone diet gives them a staggering 2,000 milligrams of calcium daily (the National Dairy Council recommends 1,200 milligrams per day), suffer one of the highest rates of osteoporosis in the world. Meanwhile, among African Bantu women, osteoporosis is virtually unknown—despite the fact that these women bear on average nine children, nurse them each two years, and ingest only about 350 milligrams of calcium a day from vegetables and legumes. The conclusion to draw, says Robbins, is not that Americans are consuming too little calcium, but rather that they are eating way too much protein. Like the Eskimo women, and unlike the Bantus, we're a nation of meat eaters. And meat, as we have already discussed, leaches calcium from our bones by making the blood so acidic that it must draw repeatedly on the buffer stored in our skeleton. Meat, alcohol, and caffeine—the holy trinity for too many Americans—all put a drain on calcium or inhibit its absorption. So does nicotine. There is no controversy in scientific circles about the biochemical, mineral-leaching activity of these substances.

Yet in typical American fashion, rather than address the root cause of the disease—by cutting way back on animal-derived protein, for example—we actually assault our overloaded systems with even more of it—in milk products—simply to get the calcium we perceive to be necessary. What adds to the perversity of this situation is our growing acknowledgment of widespread lactose intolerance.

Once milk is stripped of its osteoporosis-preventing properties, the argument for drinking it becomes mighty slim. For starters, it's got enough fat and protein in it to double the weight of a newborn calf in six weeks. That's because it was intended for cows, not humans. Cow's milk is perfect for a creature that needs to put on 100 pounds in forty-seven days. And after weaning, not even a cow drinks the stuff. We're the only creatures in the world who drink the breastmilk of another animal, and continue to do so past toddlerhood.

And finally: dairy is mucus producing, something your own mother probably recognized. If you had a cold—runny nose, sore throat, congestion, cough—she'd take you off milk, so as not to exacerbate phlegm production. That's because cow's milk has about 300 times as much casein—the same substance used as a binder in industrial strength glue—as human milk. Sure enough, the clients we see who respond dramatically to an absence of milk products are those suffering chronic phlegm conditions such as upper respiratory infections or allergies.

College student Lisa, 21, plagued with sinusitis, sought our counsel after two years of antibiotic and decongestant "therapy" had left her with gastritis, irritable bowel syndrome, a nodule on her intestine, and no relief from sinus pressure and headaches. Lisa was fed up with the sinusitis, but even more eager to get off the drugs because she could barely eat without distress. We promptly took her off dairy products, put her on vitamin and calcium supplements, and suggested eliminating wheat, a common allergen.

Lisa's condition improved measurably: no more stomach upset, and she hasn't had a single bout of sinusitis since eliminating milk products and replacing wheat with spelt, a less irritating grain.

"Used to be, if I got a cold, it went immediately into my sinuses," she recalls. "Now, I hardly get sick anymore. If I do, it doesn't last more than a day or two. I

tell all my friends, stop taking all that over-the-counter junk. You've just got to change your diet."

Anne-Marie came to us with a similar problem: inner ear infections. Except for a few weeks in July, she told us, she took antibiotics, decongestants, ibuprofen, and sedatives daily to address her chronic vertigo, sinus headaches, and ear pain and pressure. The medication wasn't working. "I'd get in my car and say a little prayer, 'Please don't let me have a dizzy spell,' " Anne-Marie recalls. "The whole thing was so annoying. I just wanted to feel well again."

She submitted to acupuncture treatments, homeopathic remedies, and a dairy-less diet—not an easy thing for Anne-Marie, whose hectic schedule and hypoglycemia made her reach for yogurt or cheese at least three times a day. Within a week, the sinus headaches disappeared. Over time, the pressure and pain in her ears subsided, and her dizzy spells all but vanished. Driving is no longer a source of stress.

THE SUGAR FIX

Anne-Marie will also tell you that in the course of getting better, a "weird" thing happened: she stopped craving chocolate.

"I was the family chocoholic," she explains. "If I had it in house, I couldn't not eat it, and I'd eat the whole thing—like a whole bag of chocolate kisses. Then I noticed, over the holidays, eating this candy-cookie I always used to love. I took a bite and had to put it down. I thought, ugh! this is too sweet, too rich. For the first time, not only didn't I crave chocolate, I found it disgusting."

Not so weird. Over and over we see our clients "cured" of sugar and chocolate cravings, either because illness provokes them into following our dietary advice or because they're able to suppress their cravings long enough (through meditation, acupressure, acupuncture, or nutritional therapy) to be released from their addiction. And addicted they are: some estimates put daily sugar consumption in this country at one-third of a pound per day per person. That figure may be rising, given the population's infatuation with "fat-free" treats—foods where fats have been effectively replaced with sugars. The stuff is everywhere, hiding as dextrose, corn syrup, high fructose corn syrup, and plain old sugar in so many products it boggles belief: there's even sugar in salt preparations! Read more labels, and it will quickly become apparent how many of us rack up 135 pounds of sugar a year.

—SWEET UNSATISFACTION—

Sugar, as the "pure" crystal we know, does not exist in nature. Cane or beet extract is chemically and mechanically stripped of its vitamins, minerals, protein, fiber, water, and original molecular structure so that when it enters the body as white sugar, all those missing nutrients—potassium, magnesium, and calcium, to name a few—must be borrowed from in-house stores, creating a nutritional deficit. This deficit in turn drives the body to crave, to want to eat in order to replenish those stolen nutrients. A craving almost anywhere in America can and will be answered with more sugary/salty/fatty stuff. Thanks to white flour and hydrogenated oils, the naked sugar therein remains naked, and the craving remains unsatisfied—setting up a spiraling cycle of compulsive eating.

Then there's sugar's effect on immunity. When we binge on simple carbohydrates, we provoke an insulin flood. All that insulin suppresses the release of growth hormone, which in turn suppresses immune function. Now remember, sugar starts out by ransacking the body's stores of nutrients; add to this the dampening effects of insulin on immunity, and it becomes obvious how sugar renders a system defenseless against acute and chronic infection.

So we were not surprised to learn that Anne-Marie had "a chocolate thing" in addition to hypoglycemia and chronic ear infections. Nor were we surprised when dietary changes cleared up both her illness and her cravings. And in the end, Anne-Marie wasn't surprised, either.

"I've always thought everybody's body chemistry is different, and balance is critical," adds Anne-Marie, a chemist by training. "Mood issues, stress, food—all those things affect chemical reactions in the body. It's just that until now, I didn't know how to get my own chemistry balanced."

FEELING LIGHT . . . IN MIND AND SPIRIT

Let us reiterate: wellness is a state of balance, whether you assess that balance biochemically or energetically. Western medicine tends to favor adjusting out-of-sync systems chemically, usually with synthesized drugs. In fact, the latest "miracle" breakthrough in treating obesity is Redux, a drug that suppresses the desire to eat by raising levels of serotonin, the brain chemical governing our sense of well-being. Individuals who are chronically deficient in this neurotransmitter behave like addicts, eating all the time to get their fix. Never mind that you can boost serotonin levels, lift depression, and quiet food cravings just by eating a diet rich in complex carbohydrates, as all our Feeling

Light participants can attest. Redux, like the antidepressant Prozac, works by simulating the serotonin "buzz" or "high" that purportedly feels so good. Neither drug addresses the fundamental problem, which is, of course, *why* people are serotonin-deficient: the carbohydrates they're eating are all the denatured, overprocessed, nutrient-barren, fatty, caloric, white foods we've talked about. People act like addicts because for all they eat, they can't ever get the vitamins, minerals, and enzymes necessary to achieve brain chemical balance.

But then, it's already clear that drugs don't cure obesity. In Europe, where Redux has been in use for some years, those with 35 percent excess body weight drop at most only 5 to 10 percent—and that's on constant drug therapy. Opponents of Redux point out that not only is it minimally effective but it's also possibly neurotoxic.

In our minds, this only serves to underscore how vital it is to treat weight problems, or any other health imbalance, holistically, instead of zeroing in on one physiological factor.

> *School counselor Mary Lynn joined our program because she was hooked on food and antidepressants, having survived eighteen years of an abusive marriage and a recent divorce. Her therapist had put her on Prozac, and when Mary Lynn complained that its effects were fading, he doubled the dosage. While it definitely helped her feel better able to cope, Mary Lynn didn't want to have to rely so heavily on medication to get her through her day. Also, she continued to seek solace in food. Finally, she said, she just didn't have any "oomph."*
>
> *That has all changed. Since adopting our complex-carbohydrate-intensive diet, Mary Lynn has succeeded*

in lowering her antidepressant dosage. But because Feeling Light is more than an eating plan, it doesn't merely adjust serotonin levels. What Mary Lynn reports is "a lightness of spirit," which has allowed her, for the very first time, to cherish herself—and quit sabotaging her health with compulsive eating. "The program's helped me get to the root of why I overeat, so now I see those binges coming," she says. "And I can ward them off, because I've tapped into this de-stressing system." She'll fix herself a cup of hot water with a calming flower essence; just the act of sitting and sipping it, she says, makes her pause and resist "grabbing whatever food I saw." She practices the stretching, breathing, and meditative exercises we've shown her. And with the acupuncture treatments she receives weekly, and the acupressure she applies to herself, Mary Lynn is no longer goaded by an insatiable appetite.

"I don't drag myself through the day anymore—and just getting dressed used to be an unhappy prospect," she observes. "I think it's made my job easier, both at school and here at home. I definitely have a better attitude. In fact, for probably the first time in my life, I feel good about myself."

THE LIFE RAFT REFLEX

Admit it: all this is very convincing, but part of you is still afraid to take a pass on the conventional sources of protein and calcium. And perhaps years of dieting have conditioned you into thinking that the last thing you want to load up on is bulky fiber and complex carbohydrates.

That makes you pretty much like everybody else we see, except that you're perhaps not as ill, or at least the only sign of illness you see is what you read on the bathroom scale. You're probably a lot like Lisa, who remembers thinking, when we said no more dairy, *What the hell am I going to eat?*

Practice any activity three times a day since infancy, and that activity becomes habit. More than a habit, actually: It becomes second nature, particularly if it's an activity as vital as eating. So even if standard American fare isn't good for you long term (and you're conscious of that, if even vaguely), chances are you're not going to let go of that habit easily. Besides, it's all you've got, so who would blame you for clinging to it? Very few people jump off a life raft, inadequate though it may be for the long haul, unless they see land and can safely swim to it.

We're going to talk about the kinds of food that will provide you safe haven. We'll show you how you're going to get to that terra firma, stroke by stroke. But as with any new adventure, it helps to unburden yourself of your past. In the next chapter, we'll discuss how to shed the baggage that may be preventing you from taking the plunge. We're going to get you to leave that life raft behind forever.

CHAPTER FIVE

Detoxification

The Cleansing Fast

Λre you toxic?

Think for a moment. Think about some of your minor indulgences, the tiny ones you commit daily. We're referring to the Equal and Cremora in your coffee, the mayonnaise in your sandwich, the Hamburger Helper you mix up for the kids and wind up eating yourself. The soda, diet or otherwise, you sip all day. Or the cookies and milk you eat standing over the sink, just before bed.

We all have our good days and bad days.

But now think of some of your worst excesses. You know: that time you pulled off the highway for coffee and ate a half dozen glazed doughnuts, or stopped at a diner for a family-sized serving of onion rings and a Coke. Those parties where you spent three hours grazing on Brie-smeared crackers, chips slathered in dip, stuffed mush-rooms slippery with butter, and little hot dogs blanketed in puff pastry. The business dinners where you overdid the prime rib. The weddings where you wallowed in baked Alaska. Happy Hours you spent awash with frozen margaritas. Saturday picnics where you pigged out. Sunday brunches that lasted till three o'clock. Monday night football with the guys, or Tuesday night gourmet club with the girls. Birthday bashes. Thanksgiving feasts. New Year's Eve blow-outs.

Nor is it just what you've *ingested:* consider the nicotine or passive smoke, the household dust, the industrial grime, the airborne lead, the unseen radon, the formaldehyde in carpets, the pesticides outdoors, the cleaning agents in-doors, and countless other carcinogens you've absorbed or inhaled every day.

Now—if you can bear it—add it all up. The everyday sins, the occasional extravaganzas. Even if you're not carrying around your crimes in the way of extra poundage, or a degenerative disease, or a chronic ailment, the toxic residue of all that you've put in your body day after day, year after year, is staggeringly oppressive.

It's a wonder the EPA hasn't targeted you. You're a toxic waste dump.

And if saturated fat, refined sugar, excessive animal protein, chemical additives, preservatives, colorings, caf-feine, pesticide residue, antibiotics, growth hormones, heavy metals, acid rain, and—dare we overlook it?—*stress* haven't yet caught up with you, you can be sure they will. We've got the cancer, heart disease, diabetes, and osteo-porosis statistics to prove it.

WIPING THE SLATE CLEAN

So. Wouldn't it be great to just *start over*?

Wouldn't you love to just be born all over again, washed clean, or purified of all this gook that's clogging, calcifying, or poisoning your system?

So strong, and so pervasive is our desire to be cleansed, renewed, or given a second chance that we'll spend $3,995 for a week at a spa, or $395 for a weekend retreat, or $39.95 for a few days' worth of meal replacements. We will pay, essentially, to be deprived—deprived of food, of stimulus, of stress, of choices. And in some instances, the therapy works: we feel better. Or at least, we feel like feeling better is possible.

We can offer you an alternative.

Our detoxification program can be done anytime. You don't have to drop out of your life or leave town. You needn't invest in tapes, gurus, loose clothing, or literature. You don't need to consult a doctor to undertake this, although, if it'll make you feel more confident, we suggest you do. Our program is safe and appropriate for virtually everyone. By the end of it you'll be cleansed. You'll be renewed. You'll have more energy, and you'll get more vitamins and minerals out of every healthful morsel you put in your mouth, so that your body will have more defenses against the ravages of modern life. And you'll feel lighter.

Because you will be lighter.

How will this cleansing be accomplished? By stopping new poisons from entering. By giving your vital digestive organs a rest. And by allowing your organs of excretion— the skin, the kidneys, the liver, and the bowels—to do their job thoroughly.

*   *   *

In a word, you're going to fast.

WHY FAST?

When you get well, weight will no longer be an issue. But to get well, you've got to undo the effects of years of toxic buildup. Food that overloads your system isn't digested; undigested food isn't passed; unpassed food accumulates as intestinal sludge and adipose tissue (fat, we call it). Poisons get stored in the liver, until the liver gets so overloaded that it spills them into the bloodstream.

So to get well you've got to flush out the fat and the poisons. You've got to give your liver and kidneys a chance to catch up on their workload, and then a rest so that their tissues can rejuvenate. You've got to scrub the bowel walls of hardened plaques, undigested proteins, fatty deposits, and chemical fallout. Once that's accomplished, the mucosal cells lining the intestines can readily absorb the nutrients you're going to start ingesting. You'll heal, and in healing, you won't be prone to the cravings and imbalances that drove you to eat too much of the wrong things and wind up in your current condition.

Weight isn't always the red flag signaling toxic overload. Many people we see complain of being tired all the time. That's because digesting and storing food that can't be assimilated or passed is a very taxing, enervating endeavor for your body. You feel chronically exhausted because you're diverting vital energies to a relentless, losing battle. Stress and exhaustion then leave you vulnerable to infection: disease gets a toehold because all your defenses are preoccupied, fighting an enemy you keep introducing.

Fasting is going to give you energy, get you well, and keep you from getting sick. And in the process, you'll lose weight. The more you have to lose, the more dramatic the effects of a fast.

WELLNESS AND WEIGHT LOSS

But isn't fasting bad for you?

We like to cite the example of a sick animal, infant, or child. What do they all do when they're fighting a viral or bacterial pathogen? They stop eating. Instinctively, they know that in order to fight off the invasive infection, they're going to need all the energies they can rally. Digesting and processing food is an energy expense they literally cannot afford. In giving the organs of digestion a rest, they can allocate those freed-up energies to fortify the front line. When they're well again, they'll eat.

And yet our response, invariably, to our child, baby, or pet during this fast is one of fear. We see their not eating as a part of the illness. We fail to perceive that fasting is one of the tools the body employs in order to heal itself.

Unfortunately, as we get older, we lose touch with the instincts that govern early behavior. We don't listen to what our bodies are telling us; on the contrary, when we're sick, we foist food upon ourselves, fearful of any lapse in nourishment. Additionally, we have our well-meaning friends, family members, and doctors advising us to eat. Little wonder fasting has come to be associated with desperate dieting and illness instead of with healing, wellness, and rejuvenation.

Fasting is an excellent way to tune back in to the body's instructions. It's also a time-honored means of tuning in to our spiritual voice: since the beginning of recorded history, men have fasted in order to cleanse their souls and heal themselves of physical, emotional, and mental disease. Fasting endures in all the world's major religions as a spiritually enriching ritual, one intended to quiet all the body's appetites so that peace might prevail and a new beginning might be possible.

For our clients, fasting is something of a jump start to our program, because nothing sheds pounds faster or establishes the mind-set of wanting to get clean and stay that way. Even a mild cleansing, with modest weight loss, is sometimes all the spark clients need to embark on the rest of Feeling Light with conviction and enthusiasm, simply because they feel so much lighter, so much more energetic. In fact, while weight loss can be the most dramatic, most measurable, most visible side effect of detoxification, other benefits we've documented include:

- Decreased appetite
- Increased energy
- Better peristalsis, no more constipation
- Fewer headaches
- Less joint and muscle pain
- Sounder sleep
- Cravings for healthy foods
- Greater commitment to healthier eating
- Lower blood pressure
- Spiritual "centeredness"
- Clearer, more focused thinking
- Fewer gastrointestinal complaints

Perhaps for all these reasons, fasting accounts for the astounding fact that people who give themselves periodic digestive "rests" tend to live longer. One study in laboratory mice which were regularly restricted to brief, water-only fasts showed a 40 percent increase in life span. Just eradicating all the poisons our liver accumulates, stores, or vents into the bloodstream and tissues would surely add a couple of years. But cleansing the bowel of the putrefied food lining its walls, inhibiting absorption of vital nutrients—that's where we believe that the process of healing and rejuvenation really begins.

SO WHY DON'T MORE PEOPLE FAST?

I'm afraid. I don't think I'm cut out for this.

Andrew, 51, an attorney and the son of a physician, admits that, although the idea of a cleansing always appealed to him, he was afraid to try it. And it is a scary notion, if all you can equate it with is starvation. Many people make that equation because the most famous fasters—political leaders, political protesters—have used starvation and our instinctive fear of it to provoke drastic change or action.

But let us point out that fasting is *not* starvation. Political fanatics and those with severe eating disorders *ignore* what their bodies are telling them, whereas we're suggesting you pay close attention to that compelling voice.

In normal fasting, true hunger doesn't kick in until all the toxins are passed and the body has exhausted its supply of highly combustible calories—those found in fat tissue, when carbohydrates are absent. Anyone who's ever fasted can attest to the fact that after a day or two of adjustment, the body goes into a period of quietude and healing. When detoxification is completed, the body demands what it needs, loud and clear. True hunger signals it's time to quit the fast, long before the body resorts to burning muscle tissue or protein for fuel.

Other than starvation, people fear failure. Universally, our clients voiced disbelief in their ability to fast. *If I could stop eating, I wouldn't be overweight in the first place!* Or: *I'm hungry all the time! How can I possibly last a day without eating!*

That may be what you're thinking, but consider what may not be so obvious:

▲ Making food choices throughout the day can be agonizing, enervating, and rife with temptation and failure, as any dieter knows. Having no choices to make can be very liberating, in terms of time, energy, and mental preoccupation.

Debbie, a 34-year-old occupational therapist who had failed at Optifast, at Weight Watchers, and at every fad diet that hit cable TV, succeeded at our seventeen-day fruit and vegetable detoxification, losing seventeen pounds and emerging with a very different sense of what her body needed to function.

"It was easy!" she insists. "Frankly, it was a relief not to have to think about eating, about what I could put in my mouth or what I should. I actually felt like I had more energy, and more time, because there was less mental focus on food and less time caught up in meals."

▲ One of the big payoffs of fasting even for a day or two is that you will reset your "hunger" drive. What amazed Debbie after she'd completed the fast and had begun eating again, was how little she really needed to feel nourished and full.

Nancy, a 45-year-old gym teacher, similarly stunned herself by finding satisfaction in a piece of fruit for breakfast, in a simple salad for lunch. "I'm not doing 'the food groups' anymore," she says. "I've learned I don't need the toast and the glass of milk with my cantaloupe at breakfast, because I'm simply not that hungry—and it's the fasting that's taught me I can eat this way."

Cravings and chronic hunger are often a result of the toxins you're harboring and the imbalance they set up. Getting rid of those toxins and giving your gastrointestinal tract a break will literally give you the clean slate you need to get back in touch with true hunger and lower your threshold for satiation. You can then supplement with the assurance that the essential nutrients your body may be lacking will be taken up where needed.

▲ When you put into practice all the components of Feeling Light, you'll be mentally, spiritually, and physically armed and ready to embark on a fasting adventure to reset your food needs and desires. Andrew, who surprised himself by sticking to water for three days, attributes his success to the meditation, the daily affirmations, and the Tai Chi that are all part of Feeling Light.

If you don't feel you're ready, think about a time in the future when you'll find it easier. Make plans for it—and work toward it.

BUT CAN *I* DO IT?

Part of succeeding at a fast lies in the realization that *you* determine what's appropriate for you—whether it's one day or twenty, whether it's water or juices, whether it's fruit and vegetables or grains.

"I chose to do the three-day water fast," says Andrew, "because no one pressured me. There was no coercion. It was just that after the meditative exercises, this was the next logical step for me."

That's an essential tenet of Feeling Light: We can give you the tools, but which ones you decide to use and when you decide to use them are entirely up to you. It's possible to detox with herbs, supplements, flower essences, Tai Chi, and a diet rich in fiber, minerals, vitamins, and essential fatty acids. In fact, if you're suffering from diabetes, true hypoglycemia, kidney disease, anemia, or severe weakness, don't fast. Nor is fasting appropriate for children, for the elderly, and for pregnant or nursing women. It's absolutely inappropriate for those with eating disorders like anorexia.

But if you're not being treated for chronic disease or acute ailments, then fasting can be a powerful weapon in your arsenal against weight, disease, and degeneration—a weapon always at your disposal. You've got to:

- pick the right time;
- pick the right fast;
- know what to expect;
- know when to quit;
- and know how to come off the fast.

We'll tackle each of these in turn.

THE BEST OF TIMES, THE WORST OF TIMES

Don't fast during the holidays. When you're assaulted not only with food but also with social pressures to eat, it's decidedly the wrong time to detox. Ditto for other events where food is the social medium and celebration: weddings, bar mitzvahs, anniversaries, confirmations, baptisms. After these events, however, you may have not only the social hiatus but also the incentive to fast, having indulged to the point where you're literally sick and tired.

Some seasons lend themselves to fasting better than others. We find it much easier, even pleasant, to fast in the spring, when we can walk outside and revel in the distractions of color and scent. There's something about the renewal going on around us that strengthens our commitment to a renewal within ourselves. Summer, too, is ideal because heat dampens our appetite and our desire to cook or prepare meals—and because when coming off the fast a wealth of seasonal fruits and vegetables awaits our savoring. For some, autumn is so evocative of a new school year, with all its promise of new projects and renewed application, that fasting is merely an extension of "turning over a new leaf." (For more guidance on when to schedule a cleansing, see our final chapter.)

When we feel in the need of a cleansing, it may simply be a matter of choosing a weekend where we can be relatively free of obligations or distractions, or choosing a week where we can be assured job stress will be minimal. During periods of tremendous emotional upheaval, many of us tend to eat or want to eat; fasting can be part of our healing process once things have calmed down or been resolved.

But the time for detoxification is right when you are ready, whether because you're desperate to initiate physical change or because you've reached a point where fasting, as Andrew says, is the next logical step. Winter or summer, Thanksgiving or spring break, if you're psyched to fast, then we urge you to listen to that urge.

WHICH FAST IS RIGHT FOR YOU?

That depends on your experience, your commitment, your preparedness, your lifestyle, and the degree to which you need to detox. Most people we've coached do best by starting small. The confidence and lightness they feel from a one-day cleansing in turn prepares them for a fast of longer duration and more dramatic results.

Mono-food Cleansing

Pick a day (we like Monday) and limit yourself to plain brown rice, brown basmati rice, or white basmati rice.

Cook it with a dash of sea salt and season with sesame seeds or sesame salt (*gomashio*). We find it easiest to have prepared a pot of rice the night before, and reheat portions as we hunger for them. Eat as much brown rice as you want, but drink plenty of water—preferably distilled water, although spring or mineral water is also acceptable. Steam-distilled water, which is available in any supermarket, is water in its purest form—no minerals, no chemicals, no additives of any type—so it truly gives your body a rest.

Sounds pretty easy, huh? It is. You can do this. You can do this every week. There's no deprivation, no gnawing hunger pangs. In fact, if it's working well for you, consider adding days.

Brown rice is nutritious and satisfying. But you might just as easily choose a fruit or a vegetable and stick with it for a day, or three days, or a week. (It may help to start by telling yourself you're only going to commit to one day; once that day's behind you, you'll find yourself excited about embarking on the next. By telling yourself you can always stop, it becomes easier and easier to add days.) Just about any one fruit—grapes, watermelon, apples, etc.— eaten exclusively constitutes a cleansing, as does a raw vegetable—carrots, celery, peppers, and the like. If your body absolutely craves a more complex carbohydrate, have brown rice for dinner. That's not failure. Everybody is different, and a fast will work for you if you give yourself some options.

Some of our clients, for instance, do a **Feeling Light Smoothie** (recipe in Chapter Seven, Super Nutrition) cleansing instead of rice or fruit or vegetables. They'll start each day with it, and then drink water the rest of the day— or they'll alternate sips of Smoothie with water throughout the day. It's a great way to feel your way into fasting. We repeat: if it works for you, meaning you can stick with it, then it's right for you.

Juice Cleansing

Maybe you're noticing some nice changes since incorporating the one-day-a-week rice-only or fruit-only fast. You're moving your bowels more often, more easily. You're feeling pared down, stronger, more confident. You're probably ready for a juice fast—the essences of fruits or vegetables, minus the bulk. The virtue of such a fast is that the juicing process does all the work your stomach normally does. You'll be getting the vitamins (and minerals, if it's vegetable juice) without taxing your system.

For starters, try apple juice, and nothing but, for a day. We prefer natural, fresh-pressed, organic, unfiltered apple juice, but even Apple & Eve will do. In fact, **any pure juice** can be substituted for apple juice; avoid pulpy or acidic juices such as orange or tomato, however. When you've succeeded for a day's duration, build up to three to five days.

Alternatively, try a day or more of clear liquids such as lemon squeezed in water, herbal tea (e.g., dandelion root tea, Pau d'arco, red clover tea, alfalfa tea), green tea, black tea, or a variety throughout the day.

Vegetable juices can be just as effective, and if you've got a juicer, you may make your own (such as carrots, beets, parsley, seeded cucumber, zucchini, or celery—separately or in any combination). For an excellent gastrointestinal tonic, try juicing raw cabbage. Drink it immediately—it's not very pleasant if it sits around. Other **"green" drinks** (refer to Chapter 7), all of them terrific blood purifiers, may be substituted in lieu of a fruit or vegetable juice once a day.

During the colder months, a hot vegetable broth can

be more soothing than cold juice. An extremely healing decoction you can substitute for juices or other clear liquids consists of:

**3 carrots
2 celery stalks
2 beets
half a head of cabbage
quarter of a bunch of parsley
quarter of an onion
half a clove of garlic**

Combine the ingredients in a pot and cover with water. Simmer the vegetables for 20 minutes and then strain them out. Drink three to five cups of this juice or broth each day for three to five days.

Sticking to fruit juice, vegetable juice, vegetable broth, or clear liquids for three to five days will optimize tissue cleansing and rejuvenation. Don't take any nutritional supplements other than the green drinks derived from chlorophyll products, as supplements are best tolerated and absorbed in the presence of food. Any liquid fast you choose can be repeated up to five times a year. (See our final chapter for help on scheduling your detoxes.)

Water Cleansing

Fasting, in its purest form, means subsisting on **water** alone. There is nothing quite like three days of water to give your body a total rest and recalibrate all gastrointestinal and metabolic meters. Such a fast will provoke your body to burn fat faster, since fat stores are burned only in the absence of carbohydrates.

If you're a seasoned faster, it won't take more than a

day before your organs settle down and stop clamoring for attention. Still, we advise you to "cool down" your metabolic furnace for two days before limiting yourself to water. Eat lightly: cooked vegetables and rice are best. For your last meal the evening before the fast, stick to raw fresh fruits or raw or lightly steamed vegetables. On Day One of the fast, drink distilled water only, and do not take any supplements of any kind. On Days Two and Three, spring or mineral water may be substituted, but distilled is preferable.

At the end of Day Three, take two small- to medium-sized apples, quarter them, and let them sit out until they turn brown (this increases the natural pectin, a soothing agent for the digestive system). Eat them slowly. We promise you these will be the best apples you've ever tasted!

The 17-Day Detox

If you're coming off a three-day water fast, there's simply no better time to launch our seventeen-day cleansing program. For one thing, your system won't be ready for anything heavier than vegetables and fruits. But to achieve a truly clean slate upon which to build new, lifetime eating habits, there's nothing like a clean break from the old habits. The seventeen-day diet of raw fruits and vegetables, following on the heels of three days of water, is just that: a total departure from habits that have imprisoned you in extra poundage.

For breakfast, start with a smoothie—the Feeling Light Smoothie detailed in Chapter 7, Super Nutrition, is ideal (made with juice instead of soy or rice milk), but any combination of fruits may be pureed frozen or with ice in a blender. Or liquefy vegetables in a juicer. Lunch and dinner can be a huge salad, dressed lightly with lemon juice, safflower or olive oil, mustard, vinegar, or tamari. Spring and mineral water should be consumed as needed, alter-

nated with any of the liquids we've described in the pre-
ceding cleansing programs. Now that you're eating, you
may resume taking all supplements, including psyllium
husks or flaxmeal for scrubbing the intestines. Again, see
our chapter on super nutrition.

One of our clients reports that being limited to fresh
fruits and vegetables made her see the produce section of
the supermarket in a whole new light. Having no need to
run off to the other aisles, she was obliged to study the
options—and was amazed at how many "new" items
caught her eye. "I was trying things I'd never even *seen*
before," she says. "It was like a whole new world opened
up, one with tremendous variety. I'd look at my cart and
it was full of nothing but fruit and vegetables!"

You may feel a craving for something *cooked* during
this detox, but hang in there. Raw fruits and vegetables are
especially effective in cleansing, healing, and weight loss
because of the enzymes released from the raw produce—
enzymes that cooking destroys. Raw produce will literally
"melt away" the fatty wastes stored in fat cells and tissues
and restore depleted enzymes. In fact, an enzyme deficiency may be why some people are overweight in the first
place, because without them, food cannot be adequately
metabolized, and winds up being stored as fat.

After seventeen days, you'll continue eating in the
same manner, but you may lightly steam the vegetables or
stew the fruit. In addition:

Week One: Add a whole grain, such as brown rice, or a
    whole grain bread.
Week Two: Introduce nuts, seeds, beans, and legumes.
Week Three: Fish and chicken may be added.
Week Four: Add, if you must, pork and beef.

If you bracket the seventeen-day program with the water
fast and this slow reintroduction of proteins, you will have

— FASTING AT A GLANCE —

FALL	WINTER
3 days of apples or apple juice	3–10 days of brown rice or 3–5 days of vegetable broth
SPRING	SUMMER
3–10 days of brown rice and spring water; gomashio on rice is optional. or 3–10 days of raw fruits and vegetables	17 days of raw fruits and vegetables

accomplished a six-week detoxification. A cleansing of this magnitude won't be necessary but once or twice a year.

ENHANCING THE HEALING

- It's important to get your lymph moving so that vented poisons will be removed from the bloodstream and excreted. A lymphatic massage, or regular "rebounding"—such as jumping on a trampoline—is an excellent way to rev up circulation and speed the toxins on their journey out of the body.
- Dry-brush your skin in the shower before turning the water on. Your skin is the largest organ of elimination, often referred to as the "third kidney." It's the first place where toxins surface. Use a natural bristle brush, and brush your entire body in strokes that aim toward the heart: ankles to knees, knees to hips, wrists to el-

bows, elbows to shoulders, lower back to shoulder blades. You'll enhance your circulation, hastening the purification of the blood. And you'll flake off dead skin with its load of leached out toxins.

- Take soaking baths and long showers.
- "Broom" your intestines. On the 17-day fast, mono-fasts, or during the weeks you're coming off a fast, be sure and take supplemental dietary fiber such as psyllium husk or flaxmeal, as we discuss in our chapter on supplements. This indigestible fiber acts like an internal bristle brush, scrubbing at the hardened plaques and layers of sludge clinging to the intestinal walls.
- A sauna, if you've got access, can be a terrific aid to cleansing the body of impurities. **Do not use the sauna during any of the liquid-only fasts.**

WHAT TO EXPECT

As your body expels its toxic tenants, you may experience any or all of the following symptoms:

- headache
- muscular aches
- weakness
- light-headedness
- slow-motion feeling
- stomach rumbling
- stomach cramping
- loose bowel movements
- a cessation of bowel movement

This is all utterly normal, particularly during the first day or two of a cleansing regimen. You're in a state of transition, where layers of poisons or plaques that haven't been disturbed for months, or even years, are coming unmoored from the colon, the blood vessels, the liver, and the skin. Prior to exodus, they can make you feel uncomfortable. Indeed, this discomfort is your strongest indication that detoxification is taking place.

Missing food, or wanting food, is a feeling that will abate within a day or less as your system quiets down. Many of our clients report a kind of euphoria setting in once some of the symptoms described above disappear: they feel super attuned, energetic, sensorily sensitive . . . and free of the burdens they've spent years accumulating.

COMING OUT OF A CLEANSING PERIOD

Discipline, oddly enough, isn't usually an issue *during* a fast. It's when the cleansing is over that you've got to exercise restraint. Psychologically, you may be telling yourself you've earned a big meal. Physically, hunger—true hunger—has returned, so that food that may have looked or smelled repulsive during the fast now holds a promise of utter pleasure.

Your stomach, endocrine system, and intestines have been resting; don't give them a rude awakening. Raw fruits, smoothies, broths and light soups, vegetables, and sprouts will be your best bets, ingested slowly, chewed or savored thoroughly. Don't pile it on: plan on grazing and sipping all day rather than eating three regular meals. Gurgling, cramping, gas, or nausea are all signals to cut back or slow down. Remember, your stomach has shrunk, and your colon is as pink as the new skin revealed beneath a scab.

Coming off a fast you're going to feel like a snake that's shed its skin: you're free of that nasty baggage you've been dragging around—inside and out—and you look and feel *newer*. You've done it! Now you can check it off that mental list of "shoulds" you carry around, and start cataloguing all the changes for the better.

Rejoicing in the New You

Feeling Light participants who have fasted report they now know what it feels like to have a furnace that burns fuel efficiently instead of one that barely smolders despite continual stoking. They're amazed at how much quicker food moves through their system, and how much more energy they get out of it.

Debbie remembers when she reached the last weeks of the two-and-a-half-month detox. She'd been looking forward to bringing fish and chicken back into her diet. But when she tried to eat these proteins, she found she'd lost her taste for them.

"The fast definitely reset the way I feel about food—about protein, and about fat especially," she comments. "Before the fast, at least fourteen of every twenty-one meals was meat of some kind; now, it's never more than three, because I just don't feel good after a heavy meal."

She's surprised to find her appetite for food suppressed; for exercise, it's heightened. "I have a lot more energy now," she insists. "I'm not tired at three in the afternoon anymore, the way I used to be every single day. And I sleep a lot better."

Nor are the effects of fasting strictly physical. Fasters also report a heightened state of awareness, a keener sense of smell, and—coming off the fast—the ability to savor the simplest of foods. Cravings for sweet or fatty foods have become sharp aversions. Fasters come to understand just what their relationship to food is—why they put what they put in their mouths. And they enjoy a tremendous confidence boost—both because they've succeeded where they were certain they would fail, and because in succeeding, they lost weight.

"It's like suddenly learning you can run five miles," says Amy, 41, a school administrator. "Your body knows just what to do: you can almost see and feel your liver cleaning itself out. And it's not just that: you look better, like you've been working out, because you've lost weight and your muscles show."

If you've fasted along the lines we've suggested, chances are you're much more in touch with what makes you eat— what hunger is, what you hunger for, and *what you no longer hunger for*. Fasting makes you an expert at decoding the urges you feel. Eating is no longer blind ritual, no longer the sort of knee-jerk response to a time of day or a period of stress. You eat when you need fuel, and you stop eating when you feel full. Eating after fasting, says Amy, "is a very deliberate act: you eat only because you really, really want to and need to. That clean feeling is something you don't want to undo—kind of like not wanting to wear new shoes outside because you don't want to get them scuffed."

After a cleansing fast, you'll find that eating—for perhaps the first time in your life—is no longer a tightrope exercise, with guilt on one side and torment on the other. So attuned are you to what your body really needs and wants—broccoli, or a ripe pear, or a bowl of pasta—that satisfaction is easy and guiltless. You will be free to heed your instincts. And they won't mislead you.

PART THREE

Go!

CHAPTER SIX

What Should I Eat?

Foods That Heal

The whole idea behind Feeling Light can be reduced to one pearl of wisdom: eat the healthiest foods you can, whenever you're hungry, and stop when you're full.

Simple, right?

Hardly. If you knew what to eat, when to eat, and how to stop eating, then there wouldn't be a 30-billion-dollar diet industry and you wouldn't be reading this book.

You can't eat moderately because you're out of balance. When you're out of whack—physically, emotionally, bio-chemically—the voice of regulation is drowned out by the voices of need. When you're not getting what you need, you can't stop craving. When you can't stop craving, you can't stop eating.

And *what* you're eating, as we've noted, is only making this vicious cycle more vicious.

Nobody, nowadays, really knows what to eat. None of our clients is quite sure what constitutes a healthy diet when they come to us for help. Rebecca, the disciple of the all-protein diet, ate cottage cheese for breakfast, tuna for lunch, and six egg whites for dinner for six months. Madeline, convinced that calories were the culprit behind her weight problem, has for years judged the healthfulness of everything she put in her mouth by the number it was assigned in a little booklet. Suzanne, certain that all fat is unhealthy, makes counting fat grams and figuring fat percentages a daily observance. Carol is watching her sugar intake, which in her mind translates into soda with NutraSweet and coffee with Equal. Emily is measuring every milligram of sodium she ingests. Cheryl believes she has a sensitivity to carbohydrates. Caroline thinks bread and pasta are fattening.

When each week another fitness or fatness book comes out with a different gospel, it's virtually impossible to know who's right and who's wrong. Fat is bad, we're told—*but eat more olive oil.* Limit your intake of cholesterol, we read—*but eat more fish.* Beware of starchy foods, we hear—*but eat more pasta.* Cut back on dairy foods, we're advised—*but be sure and get enough calcium.* Who can make healthy choices when Healthy Choice is the brand name of a TV dinner, granola bars are made with Oreos, and yogurt is blue and orange? Little wonder the well-intentioned dieter fails! When expert counsel is contradictory, and buying food is more bewildering than brain surgery, there's no joy in trying to eat "healthy."

Let's acknowledge the obvious: eating is a sensual

pleasure, an act we get to indulge in three times a day, day in and day out. Any diet that denies us this pleasure is doomed. Any diet that restricts foods to an accepted few dooms the dieter to the kind of monotony that leads to malnutrition, rather than weight loss. No human being we've ever met can diet according to deprivation and succeed; no one in our experience has ever achieved a moderate weight by taking extreme measures. Success lies in balance, in eating a modicum of a variety of foods.

So we're going to spell out the *kinds* of food you should eat. Rather than give you a detailed list of approved and nonapproved foods—the kind of "diet" you can live with for, oh, maybe two weeks—we'll arm you with the information you need to make healthy choices for satisfying meals for the rest of your life.

BREAKING THE FAST

Okay. It's the dawn of a new day. You've cleansed your body of toxins and set your mind on the salvation of your biochemical soul. You're envisioning the new you. You're going to put only good, healthy, clean food into this vehicle carrying you through life.

But it's time for breakfast, and you're hungry. What can you eat?

We don't believe in skipping breakfast, or replacing it with an "instant" milk shake that pretends to offer nutrition in place of food. However, after years of consulting with clients who have trouble getting off to a good start, we can suggest a quick, tasty concoction that satisfies not only your body's craving for fuel but also its need for minerals, vitamins, and protein so that you don't suffer cravings later in the day for any food that will knock you off course. We call this breakfast-in-a-blender the **Feeling**

Light Smoothie. (Because it's full of essential nutrients, you'll find the recipe in the next chapter, Super Nutrition.)

For many of our participants, the Smoothie is all the breakfast they want.

Emily, 44, a social worker and educator, swears by it because "it starts me out on the right foot. If I have a sweet muffin, then it's kind of like saying, 'this day's been blown,' and I may as well give up trying to eat right."

Almost all agree that it's the most satisfying breakfast of all the options we discuss, carrying them well past the dreaded coffee-hour-of-weakness into lunchtime.

Yet for a few, either because they find the green color off-putting or because they want to sit down to a more conventional meal—or because they're simply not ready to transform their diet—we offer the following suggestions:

whole grain cereal, with soy milk, rice milk, or apple juice
    grape-nuts
    Nutri-Grain Raisin Bran
    Shredded Wheat
    oatmeal
    cream of wheat or rice
    nine-grain cereal
    muesli
OR organic, whole grain baked goods, such as
    whole wheat waffles
    whole wheat English muffin
    whole wheat bagel
    multigrain or whole grain bread
OR eggs (if you must; no more than once a week)

OR fresh
  bananas
  grapefruit
  melon
OR stewed prunes
AND/OR 100% fruit or vegetable juice, such as
  cranberry
  apple
  orange
  grapefruit
  carrot
  spinach
  carrot/apple
  homemade "V8"
  tomato/cucumber/parsley/carrot/celery/beet
Tea or noncaffeinated beverage, such as
  green or black tea
  herbal tea
  grain coffee substitute
  soy or rice milk*
  cup of miso
  lemon juice in seltzer or hot water
  We recommend skim milk for those of you who can't make the change to soy or rice milk. But we strongly recommend cutting out all dairy for anyone who has upper respiratory conditions such as sinusitis, bronchitis, hay fever, or asthma, or gastrointestinal problems such as constipation, diarrhea, or irritable bowel syndrome.
USE SPARINGLY—spreads and sweeteners, such as
  honey
  blackstrap molasses
  all-fruit jelly
  real maple syrup
  nut butters
  flaxseed oil

These are merely suggestions. You can add considerably to this list of options if you bear in mind the following guidelines:

- Grains are good, whole grains are better, and organic whole grains are best.
- Fruit should be fresh and pesticide-free, but dried fruit is okay, and canned fruit is better than no fruit at all.
- Freshly made juice is always best, but frozen or jarred juice is acceptable, provided it consists of nothing but juice.
- Sweeteners that occur naturally—even white sugar— are always preferable to chemical substitutes such as saccharine, aspartame (NutraSweet), or sorbitol.
- Fats or oils that are solid at room temperature should be used very sparingly. Stay away from butter on your bread until you've lost the weight, and then use it only occasionally. Don't use margarine.
- Unrefined is always preferable to refined; unprocessed is always preferable to processed, because processing destroys or strips away nutrients and typically adds coloring agents, preservatives, reconstituted vitamins, and other chemicals.
- The more perishable a food—the shorter its shelf life— the healthier it is.
- The best foods need no advertising and require little or no packaging.

FAT: WHO NEEDS IT?

You do.

All the brouhaha about fat and its evils has drowned out a critical fact. No matter what your weight, certain kinds of fat—the so-called **polyunsaturates**—have substances *essential* to health. Some scrub the arteries of dangerous plaques, lowering cholesterol and the risk of heart disease. Others have elements vital to cell growth and to the production of prostaglandins, which regulate blood pressure, heart rate, clotting, and the central nervous system. A no-fat diet is not only impracticable but also unhealthy: fat aids in the transport and absorption of many vitamins. We need fat for energy, for warmth, and to keep our nerves protected and our organs in their proper place. When fat is not available to burn, the body resorts to the protein in muscle tissue. And when protein is being used for fuel, it cannot be used for its primary function, which is to synthesize new tissue.

In short, if you're deficient in substances called **essential fatty acids (EFAs)**, you'll suffer a host of bodily plagues and go through the day with a gnawing, desperate hunger that's likely to derail you from healthful eating altogether.

Of course, as we discussed in the previous chapter, there are fats you most certainly don't need, but it's easy to remember which ones if you remember simply this: **Anything from an animal has fat you don't want. Anything from the earth—derived from plant matter, that is—has the fat you most definitely need in order to function and stay well.** Foods that are especially high in EFAs include:

All grains, including
    barley
    corn
    oats
    wheat
    rice
    millet
    rye
    spelt

Dark green leafy vegetables, including
    collard greens
    turnip greens
    beet greens
    mustard greens
    dandelion greens
    spinach
    kale
    watercress
    parsley

Nuts, such as
    chestnuts
    pistachios
    almonds
    pecans
    walnuts
    filberts
    Brazil nuts
    macadamia nuts
    hazelnuts
    cashews

Seeds, such as
    pumpkin seeds
    flax seeds
    sesame seeds
    sunflower seeds

Legumes, such as
    soybeans
    peanuts
    pine nuts

Avocados

Olives

Vegetable oils, such as
    olive
    canola

safflower
sunflower
soybean
corn
sesame

Because most of us simply don't eat enough of these foods, most of us are deficient in EFAs—a problem which can manifest itself in the following illnesses:

acne	fibrocystic breast disease
allergies	hypertension
atherosclerosis	inflammation
autoimmune disorders	lupus
bronchial asthma	multiple sclerosis
cancer	obesity
cardiovascular disease	rheumatoid arthritis
diabetes	schizophrenia
eczema	ulcerative colitis

But part of our deficiency can also be traced to the fact that EFAs are not very durable. Overprocessing destroys them, making any oil that's not cold-pressed or expeller-pressed pretty much a nonnutritive fat. Also, nuts, seeds, and the oils derived from them have a relatively short shelf life: heat, light, or oxygen can spoil them, and rancidity renders them not only devoid of EFAs but also possibly carcinogenic. In a culture habituated to once-weekly supermarket visits—or food-by-the-case shopping sprees at bargain warehouses—an unstable oil is an undesirable one. Oils that are highest in EFAs are therefore the least likely to show up on the shelves.

Certain cold-water fish are a good source of EFAs. They are:

sardines	sablefish
salmon	bluefish
albacore tuna	trout
Atlantic mackerel	mullet
Atlantic herring	bass

Many studies confirm that the oils in these fish lower levels of "bad" cholesterol while raising levels of "good" cholesterol, thereby reducing the risk of stroke or coronary. Since no one can agree on how much fish provides protection against heart disease, we'll stick with our original recommendation that you limit your meat meals (including fish) to three per week. Fish, like any other animal flesh, is an acidifying food that can disrupt body pH if consumed in excess.

Whatever the source, EFAs are your best insurance against the kind of imbalance that's making you sick, causing you to age, or skewing your weight toward extremes by making you constantly hungry. When your EFAs are in balance, you'll likely not suffer from some of the cravings that lead to weight imbalances and saturated fat excesses. In fact, **correcting an EFA deficiency will help you lose weight**: EFAs are thought to increase metabolic rate to the point where excess fat and glucose are burned away.

COFFEE BREAK?

Too many people seek relief from that draggy feeling they suffer daily by drinking coffee. "I need the boost," they tell us, apologetically. "Caffeine gets me through the morning."

Part of the beauty of a breakfast high in complex carbohydrates—whole grains or fruit—is that you won't have that hollow, shaky feeling by midmorning. Skipping breakfast out of haste or calorie-consciousness winds up being utterly counterproductive: you waste time dwelling on food, and then consume calories you instantly regret in the form of coffee-break foods—donuts, danish, muffins, buttered rolls, or bagels. And coffee itself.

In fact, some of our clients concede that in the course of a day they'll drink six to eight cups of coffee for "energy." In moderate amounts, caffeine is a proven stimulant, but because coffee is a diuretic, such a habit winds up being dehydrating, and thus fatiguing. Even decaffeinated coffee in these amounts has a deleterious effect, largely because of the chemical residue that the decaffeinating process leaves on the beans. Methylene chloride, a known carcinogen used to extract caffeine, may be present in trace amounts.

Better to switch your brew altogether. As with any habit you're trying to break, go slowly and substitute, rather than go cold turkey. One cup of coffee is better than six. One cup of decaf is better than one cup of regular coffee. **Green and black teas**—including ordinary Lipton, as well as those packaged by Celestial Seasonings and those found in Oriental markets and health food stores— are better than decaf coffee, despite the fact that they're caffeinated, because they're sources of cancer-preventing substances known as antioxidants. **Herbal teas** may be altogether a better choice, given their soothing and hydrating effects.

If these alternatives simply aren't your cup of tea, consider grain concoctions such as **Postum, Roma, Cafix, or Pero**. For a real change of pace, we recommend a cup of **miso**, readily mixed from a packet of miso (freeze-dried fermented bean paste) and eight ounces of boiled water. Similarly nutritive drinks found in a health food store include **Suma, Raja's Cup**, and **Pau d'arco**, which have the added benefit of boosting the immune system and fighting yeast infection. Water in which **roasted dandelion root** has simmered for twenty minutes makes a wonderful coffee substitute that also detoxifies your liver. **Bancha twig tea** with a touch of tamari will give a coffeelike pick-me-up. **Lemon juice in hot water** can be a refreshing change. And a cup of **boiling water with a tablespoon of blackstrap molasses**—sugar in its crudest form—is full of iron and calcium and is naturally sweet.

SWEET NEWS FOR SWEETS LOVERS

Sugarcane is not a bad source of sweeteners, *provided* they're completely unrefined: among our favorites are **blackstrap molasses** and Sucanat™, which is 100 percent evaporated sugarcane. All the minerals and vitamins remain intact, as opposed to white sugar, which actually robs the body of the minerals necessary for sucrose digestion because the refining process has stripped away those originally present in sugarcane. But there are a variety of other natural sources, some with decided advantages over even unrefined cane products.

Stevia, a liquid extracted from the stevia plant, is a noncaloric sweetener thirty times as sweet as sugar. There seems to be no downside to stevia (unless you're in the sugarcane industry): it doesn't affect blood glucose levels (good news for diabetics), it lowers high blood pressure, inhibits the growth of bacteria that causes tooth decay, and decreases cravings for other sweets or fatty foods. It's the sweetener of choice in Paraguay, China, Taiwan, Thailand, Korea, Malaysia, Indonesia, and Japan, where stevioside (a derivative 300 times sweeter than sugar) accounts for 41 percent of the market. The FDA has not sanctioned stevia's use as a sweetener, but it can be found in health food stores as a dietary supplement.

Fructose is a sugar naturally occurring in fruit and honey and is best consumed along with those sources, because all the vitamins and minerals necessary for its absorption are present. **Honey** can be a healthful sweetener, but it is no different from white sugar if it's pasteurized and filtered, so choose organic raw honey, as fresh from the hive as possible. **Rice and brown rice syrup**, similar in texture to honey, come from fermenting the grain and boiling it into syrup. **Barley malt**, in syrup and powder forms, is an excellent substitute, as it can be used in cooking and baking. **Carob molasses, carob syrup**, and **date sugar** can also stand in for cane sugar products. Or try **maple syrup** or **apple juice** in pies or desserts.

LUNCH AT YOUR DESK

Our favorite midday meals come from dinner the night before, which we make extra ample just to generate leftovers for lunch. If dinner was on the late side (and that's pretty often, it seems), we'll eat lightly then and look forward to having our "big" meal midday. The old saw about eating like a queen at lunch and like a pauper at dinner is full of contemporary wisdom, as we digest and burn a big lunch but tend to store a big dinner. If we're short on leftovers, however, and we have access to a stove, a quick lunch might consist of a **veggie burger, home-made soup, a tofu hot dog, or a pot of rice with vegetables.**

Good, healthful, tasty lunches can come out of a paper bag, too. Our more portable repertoire includes:

- tuna (hold the mayo) on whole wheat bread
- fresh fruit salad
- butterleaf salad with mandarin orange slices, sunflower seeds, and sesame oil
- taboule with lemon juice, tomato, scallions, and bean sprouts
- whole wheat pita stuffed with bell peppers, tofu, and cooked sweet potato
- brown rice with adzuki beans and gomashio
- romaine salad with tomatoes, cucumbers, and olive oil and lemon dressing
- minestrone soup and half a whole wheat bagel with all-fruit sugarless jelly
- lentil soup
- spinach salad with shredded carrots, mushrooms, and lemon-dijon dressing
- nine-grain bread with tahini (sesame butter), half a grapefruit, and romaine/arugula salad with tomatoes, cucumbers, and sesame-poppyseed dressing
- soycheese sandwich
- whole wheat bread with vegetarian bologna, lettuce, tomato, and dijon mustard
- turkey on whole grain bread with lettuce and honey mustard

GOOD, BETTER, AND BEST

Did your eyes deceive you? Was that *turkey* you saw in that sandwich we listed? Turkey, as in *lunch meat*?

As we've said before, weaning you away from meat and dairy is a slow and purposeful endeavor. If you're going to consume meat (and we'd recommend it appear in no more than three out of twenty-one meals each week), choose wisely. Organic beef is better than USDA. White meat is theoretically better than red meat, although the bacteria levels typical to most fowl make most of it as toxic as red meat is fatty. White turkey meat is better than chicken of any description.

> The idea is to move you from bad choices to good, good to better, better to best.

Regarding meats, you're best off slicing your own from a roast. If you must resort to packaged processed lunch meats, then choose carefully: there's turkey, chicken, beef, pork, salami, liverwurst, bologna, and scrapple, listed in ascending order of horror. Scrapple, headcheese, chitlins, or any variation on a compost of unknowable animal parts should not be a part of any creature's diet, let alone yours. Bologna and hot dogs barely deserve to rank above this classification, as even the non-pork, "kosher" varieties have stuff (nitrites, chiefly) in them we wouldn't feed our dog. Conventional processed meat, in fact, is likely to be preserved with nitrites, so our recommendation is to buy whole, organic deli meats, meaning *nothing* but possibly salt and/or water have been added.

With regard to cheeses, we stand by our conviction that cow's milk and products derived from it should be used only as condiments, not foodstuffs. Cheeses derived from goat's and sheep's milk, while still dairy products, would be our choice, as these tend to be lower in allergens and more closely aligned with the nutritional composition of human milk. Whatever the dairy product used, however, make sure it's *real*. Choose hard rather than soft varieties, since the softer the cheese, the higher its ratio of saturated fats. Absolutely off-limits are "pasteurized cheese food" products such as in "deli singles" or cheeses found outside the refrigerated dairy section. If it doesn't need refrigeration, comes in a jar, or exists as a powder in a cardboard box, don't go near it.

—FOODS WE WOULDN'T FEED
OUR WORST ENEMY—

- Cheez Whiz (or that nacho goo they squirt on chips at the movie theatres)
- anything made by Hormel
- yogurt that's an Easter egg color
- scrapple
- maraschino cherries
- foods made with lard
- foods made with hydrogenated oils
- marshmallow fluff
- canned spaghetti

READ THE LABEL!

One glance at the labels of any of the aforementioned items and you'd know you were dealing with toxic waste. But a lot of products are nowhere near as obvious a poor choice. You've got to read the label to know the difference between real and really chemical.

To make it easier for you to compare and make healthier choices, the FDA has made labeling consistent and easier to read. All ingredients must be listed according to their preponderance in the product, meaning the first ingredient in the list is what there's most of, and the last, what there's least of. Labeling criteria and increased public awareness have had their effect: cereal manufacturers now offer a number of brands wherein sugar is no longer the first, and therefore predominant, ingredient. Overall, the FDA's campaign has had a positive effect. The educated consumer is a choosier consumer.

But in response, manufacturers have cooked up advertising and packaging stratagems designed to lead that educated consumer astray. The most notorious is probably that "all-natural" banner bedecking everything from chips to candy bars. Natural is not necessarily healthy, as you can see just by reading a package of granola bars—they're loaded with brown sugar and tropical oils.

Then there's the "healthy" band: look in the soup aisle, and what used to be strictly Campbell's territory has expanded to include a variety of no-salt, low-salt, low-fat, "healthier" choices, including Campbell's own "Healthy Request" line of reduced-salt, lower-fat soups. Indeed, compared to their original cream of chicken soup—where salt precedes chicken on the list of ingredients—the Healthy Request version is a marked improvement. Sodium is down by half, from a staggering 890 grams (37 *percent* of your daily intake) to 480 (a "mere" 20 percent), and fat is down to a quarter of its original levels. But note what goes into the "healthy" recipe: chicken fat, heavy cream, salt, disodium inosinate, disodium guanylate, potassium chloride, and "flavor." Of course, everything's relative: in the original ("Unhealthiest Request"?), there's coloring, preservatives, and that dread "flavor enhancer," monosodium glutamate, or MSG.

By no means are we singling out Campbell's for abuse. Canning, by definition, means preserving food from bacterial breakdown via the time-honored use of salt, sugar, and/or cooking the life out of it. The nutrients left after this process are as minimal as the taste, although usually the latter is beefed up with MSG, more salt and sugar, or fat. As if that weren't enough, many canned products also include sodium phosphate, BHT, or other preservatives to ensure that the food inside lasts well into the next millennium. By the time you open the can, trace amounts of aluminum may have leached into the contents—and aluminum is thought to be one of the culprits in causing the plaques responsible for Alzheimer's.

WHAT TO BUY

Here's our advice: **don't eat anything with ingredients you can't pronounce.** Better yet, don't buy anything canned. Skip the whole aisle. In fact, pretty much every foodstuff in a bottle, jar, box, or can is a waste of time if you're seeking to maximize nutrition and minimize toxins.

Oh, but surely there are exceptions. Yes. Surely. Sardines come to mind, as does that bottle of cold-pressed virgin olive oil. The entire whole grain and bean/legume aisle is worthy of your attention, if you can find there:

white basmati rice	black turtle beans
brown basmati rice	red beans
brown rice	pigeon peas
wild rice	black-eyed peas
quinoa	split peas
buckwheat	white beans
barley	navy beans
corn	Great Northern beans
taboule	fava beans
couscous	garbanzo beans (chickpeas)
lentils	kidney beans
pinto beans	lima beans
black beans	

Among the baking staples, look for:

cornmeal
whole wheat flour
rye flour
unbleached flour

Among the pasta possibilities, the best are those made with organic ingredients. Try:

jerusalem artichoke
semolina
whole wheat
spinach

The healthiest tour of the typical supermarket happens
also to be the quickest: shop around the edges. That's because all the least processed and most perishable foods are
out there, not in among the cleaning solvents and cases of
Kool-Aid. Among the fresh fruits and vegetables, you really *don't* have to pick and choose. They're all good (and
even better if organically grown). To be sure, some produce is higher in fiber, richer in beta-carotenes, or higher
in mineral content than others. But if it's fresh and from
the earth, you can't go wrong. The more seasonal, the more
likely the produce hasn't been losing vitamin potency due
to long-distance shipping.

CRUCIAL CRUCIFEROUS

Called "cruciferous" because their flowers have four petals
resembling a crucifix, the dozen vegetables below deserve
special mention for their proven role in preventing cancer,
especially cancers of the gastrointestinal tract—the esoph-
agus, larynx, pharynx, stomach, colon, and rectum. These
vegetables all high in antioxidants (vitamins A, C, and E),
fiber, chlorophyll, and natural chemicals that prevent or
retard tumor growth.

- broccoli
- Brussels sprouts
- cabbage
    Napa
    bok choy
    celery cabbage

- cauliflower
- horseradish
- kale
- kohlrabi
- mustard greens
- radishes
     or daikon (a long white root somewhat milder in taste to radish)
- rutabaga
- turnip
- watercress

Eat at least one a day!

GIFTS FROM THE SEA

You're already eating some of them. They're hidden as thickeners, emulsifiers, and stabilizers in everything from diet yogurt and ice cream to breads, puddings, and canned goods. You're also rubbing them into your skin, painting them on your wall, and spreading them on your garden as fertilizer.

They're sea vegetables, or seaweeds, as we're accustomed to calling them, because they grow so profusely in the ocean that we have no need to cultivate them. But as weeds, they tend to get overlooked: most Americans do not appreciate what an incredible food source sea vegetables are. They're tasty in a way no land vegetable can approximate, adding a nutlike savoriness to soups, grain dishes, salads, sautes, and casseroles. They add interest, color, and texture to elevate everyday cooking into culinary art. And they are really, really good for you: all seaweeds are dense with minerals, notably calcium, iron, phosphorus, potassium, manganese, sodium, zinc, and iodine. In dulse, for example, there are *forty-three* trace minerals. Sea veggies are also concentrated sources of vitamins A, all the B complex (including B12, rarely found in the plant world), and C. They're the perfect antidote and alternative to meat and dairy, as they're high in protein without the accompanying cholesterol—in fact, sea vegetables have been shown to lower blood cholesterol levels.

For healthy nails, hair, bones, teeth, thyroid function, and digestion, sea vegetables are a dietary must. For unhealthy people—those exposed to chemotherapy or radiation—seaweeds can be lifesaving de-contaminators. For the overweight, seaweeds are useful digestion stimulants, effectively "firing up" the metabolic furnace by supplying iodine to the thyroid.

But what do I buy? What do I look for? How do I use them? Don't be intimidated! Health food stores or Oriental markets carry an assortment of dried, roasted, and, occasionally, even fresh seaweeds. Here's some guidance to arm you for your foray into the unknown:

- **Agar agar**—A gelatinlike substance that comes in flakes, bars, and granules. It's used in place of animal gelatins or cornstarch or tapioca to thicken fruit compotes, cobblers, and jellies, or to thicken sauces, soups, or even stir-fries. Agar has the advantage of being more nutritious and less disruptive on blood sugar levels than cornstarch—and it doesn't introduce an unwelcome flavor or texture.
- **Arame**—You'll find these skinny, black, curly strands precooked, so that they're dried and crumbly. Use the equivalent of a tablespoon—sort of a large pinch—in any side dish of grains or legumes; one of our favorite concoctions is brown rice and adzuki beans accented with arame. Or we saute onions, carrots, parsnips, and rutabaga, and when the vegetables are crisp-tender, we throw in the arame and a splash of tamari, stir it for

15 seconds or so, and serve over rice. Because it's mild in taste and not at all slimy, arame is a good seaweed to start with if you're skittish about incorporating sea vegetables into your cooking.

- **Dulse**—Purplish petallike leaves—like torn pieces of lettuce—are sundried so that they're soft and chewy right out of the bag. Dulse makes a great snack with a little lemon juice squeezed on it; we're also fond of it as a relish with potatoes or fish because it's got such a distinctive, intense, nutlike taste. It's a great way to boost the nourishment in soups, salads, and sandwiches, too. Soaking depletes its mineral content; just rinse it slightly before using. Try roasting dulse in a 250-degree oven so that it can be crumbled onto salads and pasta. Stir-frying is another way to incorporate it into cultivated vegetable preparations.
- **Hijiki**—This seaweed comes dried in black, bulbous blades that swell up considerably when boiled or steamed with other vegetables and grains. It's used like arame, in small amounts. But because it's not precooked, hijiki works better when used to bolster soups, rice, stews, or casseroles. Just a few small pieces will add color, seasoning, and chewiness.
- **Kelp**—If you've ever been scuba diving, you know how huge and pervasive a kelp field can be. The light brown to olive brown leaves come dried in broad, flat blades, delicately wrinkled and eroded at tips; if you buy it this way, soak it for twenty minutes, slice it up, and, using the soaking water, make a soup of it. The leaves can also be steamed or stewed with land vegetables, but more often than not, kelp finds its way into our diet as a condiment or nutritional supplement (in a powdered form, or even capsules or tablets). See our chapter on super nutrition.

- **Kombu**—We prefer this to kelp in texture and taste. It comes dried in ruler-sized blades that are slightly ruffled and wavy. Soak it for twenty minutes, cut it up, and use it along with the soaking water to make soup, or cook it with beans and rice. The texture is quite delicate, and not at all slimy; the taste is mildly sweet. Kombu has more dietary fiber than oat bran!
- **Nori**—Anyone who's ever enjoyed sushi knows nori— the black-green wrapping around the rice roll that tastes delicately salty and nutty. Nori comes dried and roasted in notepaper-sized flat sheets, which may be crumbled over food or used to roll around sticky rice. When it absorbs the moisture of the rice, it's quite chewy; straight out of the bag it's crispy enough that our kids eat it as an unadorned snack.

—FOODS THE PEOPLE AT HORMEL THINK ARE YUCKY—

- seaweeds
- veggie burgers
- veggie bologna
- tofu deli slices
- tempeh
- tofu
- soy milk

WHY SOY?

America may be the world's foremost grower of soybeans, but we're the last people on earth to reap the health benefits from this cheap, plentiful source of protein. We export the bulk of our harvest, acculturated as we are into per-

ceiving soy as a Third World protein. Despite the overwhelming evidence that our First World dietary habits are
killing us, most Americans still think of soy as an "alternative" food—a main course for vegetarians.

But soy isn't meat's second cousin: it's a better choice
in every way. Meat can cause heart disease; soy can prevent it or check its progress. Meat can leach vital minerals,
particularly calcium, from the body's stores; soy can replenish those stores with calcium, iron, and phosphorus.
Meat is high in protein, but also high in fat and cholesterol;
soy offers 50 percent more usable protein than steak, but
without the cholesterol and saturated fat (instead, it's high
in essential fatty acids). Meat is loaded with hormones,
antibiotics, and pesticides; soy is naturally organic. Meat
is expensive; soy is cheap. And soybeans are high in fiber,
one of the key antidotes to a high-cholesterol diet.

As if this weren't argument enough, soybeans abound
in phytochemicals, substances we now recognize as formidable weapons in our fight against both cancer and
heart disease. Phytochemicals have been shown to lower
cholesterol levels, protect cells from assault by free radicals, deactivate carcinogens, and boost the immune system's defenses against infection.

But to benefit from these substances, we've got to make
soy a staple of our diet, much as the rest of the world has
been doing for centuries. While some 12,000 products on
our supermarket shelves do list soy as an ingredient, typically it's in the form of "partially hydrogenated" soybean
oil—a product whose processing utterly destroys soy's
healthful properties. The good news is that tofu, tofu burgers, tofu deli slices, soy milk, and a host of other unadul-
terated soy products are among the 12,000 food items from
which to choose. Substituting soy for meat and dairy has
never made more sense—and it's never been easier.

DOES THIS MEAN SHOPPING AT HEALTH FOOD STORES?

For a lot of people today, a health food store conjures images of a dingy place where long-haired men and long-skirted women pick over bins of damaged-looking produce.

That's too bad, because nothing could be further from the truth. Where we live, health foods—organic produce, soy products, rice milks, Asian condiments, and whole grain cereals—are increasingly available at major-chain supermarkets, or they are sold in a supermarketlike setting like Fresh Fields. In strip malls everywhere we see "green" markets, organic produce markets, and Oriental or Asian markets cropping up. Farmers' markets, once available only to rural and urban populations, have infiltrated the suburbs. The original health food stores—selling everything from homeopathic remedies to bulk spices and herbs—still exist, but they cater to a clientele that defies stereotyping. Health food has gone mainstream, as pesticide scares and hormone controversies make "nutriceuticals" the buzzword of the nineties.

Of course, as more and more people "discover" health foods, more and more foods that aren't particularly healthy find their way into these stores. "All-natural ingredients" certainly sounds enticing, but under this heading fall foods loaded with sugar and saturated fat. You'll find canned goods, candy ("energy" bars), and chips (fried!), along with cow's milk (minus the hormones) and even frozen yogurt, which happens to be full of natural but unhealthy ingredients like sucrose. As always, we recommend that you read labels.

While some people go into a health food store and have to be steered away from certain foods, others—including many of our clients—are reluctant to buy anything. They're overwhelmed by the unfamiliar. They're not sure what to buy, or what brand to buy. They don't know how to cook what they buy. Their kids won't eat the stuff. They already have a lot of food in their pantry. They're so reluctant, and their excuses are so varied, that you'd think we had asked them to go stock up on plutonium.

RESTOCKING YOUR PANTRY

So let's get you started. Here's a primer on health food that's healthy, and that may or may not be available anywhere but in a health food store. If it's brands or anything else that confuses you, ask the proprietor for help. And remember: you don't need to go buy all this stuff right now, in one burst of adventuresomeness. Better to zero in on a few items, and experiment incorporating them into your everyday diet, before exploring some of the others.

- **Adzuki beans**—These small red beans with a black or white dot are among the most nutrient-packed of all legumes and will help your kidneys function better. They're especially tasty cooked with brown rice and hijiki or arame seaweed and seasoned with sesame salt (gomashio).
- **Amaranth**—A dietary staple of the Aztec Indians, this small seed packs a lot of nutritional power: it's high in calcium, iron, and the amino acid lysine. Cook it as you would rice. **Amaranth flour,** a ground version of the seed, makes a wonderful addition to pancakes and other baked goods.
- **Amazake**—Yet another tasty alternative to milk, soda, or juice. This refreshing, light beverage is a kind of rice milk prepared from a mixture of fermented sweet rice and water. You'll find it in a variety of flavors: almond is one of our favorites.
- **Buckwheat groats**—More often than not, you'll find these in grain concoctions called kasha. They're made

from whole roasted buckwheat, and they are tasty in cereals, soups, and stuffings. Kasha and bowtie pasta is a traditional Jewish dish that warms the soul and satisfies the tastebuds.

• **Bulgur**—Simply wheat that's been steamed and dried before being ground. You can cook it as you would rice, for an interesting side dish or as a bed for sauteed or steamed vegetables, or even as a breakfast cereal with dried or fresh fruit mixed in.

• **Millet**—Similar in size and shape to amaranth, millet is the cereal of choice in Asia and a staple of some of the longest-lived people in the world. It's extremely high in protein and lecithin, as well as iron, potassium, magnesium, calcium, phosphorus, certain amino acids, and vitamin B2. You'll find it in breads, or you can cook and season it as you would rice. Mixed with other grains—with buckwheat, for example—millet adds a nice, light texture and flavor. We even eat it as a breakfast cereal.

• **Miso**—Stricly speaking, miso is just fermented soybean paste. But it's an immensely versatile, nutritious staple: we drink it in hot water as a tea, we add it to soups, we blend it into salad dressings, and we add it to stir-fries. Miso comes in packets of powder for making single cups of an instant hot beverage; it also is packaged as a paste in plastic pouches or small tubs. It can be brown, tan, almost white—even reddish in color. The paste will keep in your refrigerator for months; the packets make for a highly portable pick-me-up drink at work or away from home. Very high in B vitamins.

• **Mochi**—This is sweet rice that's been pounded and then packaged in flat, scored squares. It comes in a variety of flavors, such as plain, mugwort, cinnamon, and garlic. When it's broken up into chunks and baked in a very hot oven, mochi puffs up and hollows out in the middle, allowing you to stuff each chunk with vegetables or sprouts—a terrific hors d'oeuvre. For a dip, try tahini, mustard, or a mixture of tamari, olive oil, and garlic.

- **Quinoa**—The grainlike fruit of an herb grown in the Andes. Quinoa is a complete protein. It's lighter than couscous, more flavorful, and more nutritious, with potassium, iron, zinc, and B vitamins. Mix it with grapes, sunflower seeds, and a dash of tamari and lemon for a dinner side dish. Makes a nice breakfast cereal, too. Look for **quinoa pasta,** as an alternative to semolina.
- **Spelt bread, spelt pasta**—Often used as an alternative to wheat where wheat-sensitivity is suspected, spelt is a complete protein that's also high in fiber and B vitamins.
- **Taboule**—A wheat "salad" usually sold dry and mixed with herbs. Olive oil, lemon juice, and water are added to hydrate it.
- **Tahini**—A "butter" made from sesame seeds. It's delicious as such, or incorporated into hummus. Use it on toast, muffins, crackers; a great ingredient for salad dressing, sauces, and dips.
- **Tamari**—A slow-fermented soy sauce that's lower in sodium, and richer in taste because it's naturally aged. We splash it on virtually everything we eat for a flavor boost.
- **Tempeh**—A firm, chewy rectangle of soy, derived from cooked soybeans and/or grains with a culture added. It may be sliced and sauteed, baked, or put into sandwiches.
- **Tofu**—Soy milk solidified into a semisoft white cake through the use of a mineral salt. A complete protein.

WHAT DO I FEED THE KIDS?

We hear this all the time. It's not so much a problem with adolescents, who, according to several polls, are more health-conscious in their eating habits than their parents. But grade-schoolers, under steady assault by a blitzkrieg of ads directed at their faddish sensibilities, manage to subsist on a steady diet of macaroni 'n cheese, pizza, chicken nuggets, and PB&J, all washed down with ample amounts of milk, soda, or sugary juice "drink."

They seem none the worse for wear. More to the point, say their parents, they won't eat anything else. Certainly not *tofu*.

Fine. Don't feed them tofu, at least not to start. Take whatever they're eating and un-process it. That means making macaroni and cheese with dried or fresh pasta, preferably organic (we like DeBoles), and substituting soy cheese for milk-based cheese; on pizza, Pizsoy. Replace the breaded, fried, or oil-laden nuggets with real chicken, minus the skin. Peanut butter and jelly isn't so bad, but you can make it better: Try freshly ground peanut butter and all-fruit sugarless jam on wheat or another type of whole grain bread.

Replace the cow's milk with soy or rice milk. There are many brands, some enriched with calcium, Vitamin D, and acidophilus cultures, but see which ones your kids like, and try different flavors—plain, vanilla, or cocoa. (One way to entice them is to mix up a "Banana Dream" smoothie: In a blender, combine a frozen, ripe banana with a cup of vanilla Rice Dream and a few drops of vanilla extract.) Cut out the soda altogether. Buy juice that's 100 percent real fruit juice or that doesn't add sweeteners. Bet-

ter yet, get a juicer and make your own. If the kids can get
in on the act, all the more reason to do it.

Don't make the mistake of stocking your shelves with
junk. Junk is anything heavily advertised on TV or packaged to appeal to a five-year-old. It's expensive, has virtually no nutritional value, and has been known to
adversely influence young behavior—not because kids are
hyper after eating it but because kids are hyper at the prospect of eating it. If you buy it, you'll eat it, whereas if you
don't have it around, your children will be forced to seek
alternatives, such as:

Snacks and Quickie Foods
- dried fruits *(instead of candy, but don't eat more than a few)*
    dates
    raisins
    figs
    apricots
- fresh fruits
    apples
    pears
    cantaloupes
    grapes
    strawberries
    bananas
    kiwis
- pretzels
- popcorn
- fat-free, low-salt tortilla chips *(without dyes, preservatives, or additives)*
- whole grain crackers
- soy nuts
- sesame buds
- tamari-roasted sunflower seeds

- roasted pumpkin seeds
- rice crackers
- rice/seaweed crackers
- rice cakes
- apple chips *(without dyes, preservatives, or additives)*
- sesame crackers
- Hain's carrot chips
- nuts *(raw, unsalted, or roasted—not boiled in oil)*
- freeze-dried soups
- celery sticks
- carrot sticks
- green or red pepper slices
- Barbara's cookies
- Frookies

Of course, your kids may well find unhealthful alternatives outside the home, at their friends' houses, in stores, in vending machines: worry not. You don't have to outlaw Halloween or make your kids miserable at birthday parties. Your job is not to police every morsel that passes their lips but to make good foods available and demonstrate good eating habits every meal, every day.

In fact, if you're a consistent model of good habits, there's no better way to ensure that your kids will pick up those habits in time. Rather than be a broken record they quickly learn to tune out, say nothing. Show, don't tell. Let them witness you preparing, enjoying, savoring your food. Play up the novelty of a new food item—its look, its feel, its smell. Don't beg them to be interested, and don't force them to eat it: curiosity will ultimately compel them to ask for a taste. Pretend to resist. Assure them they *won't* like it. You don't want to waste it on them; it's too good.

If indeed they don't like something they try, be neutral. Tastes change. Consistent behavior pays off. Little by little, then by leaps and bounds, you will make inroads.

And then you will have given your children a great gift—eating habits that will safeguard their health the rest of their lives.

BUT WHAT ABOUT CALCIUM?

If milk and dairy are out, how's a body to get enough calcium?

This question torments just about every woman who seeks our counsel. The brainwashing that's gone on about osteoporosis and milk is so thorough that you'd think we had suggested blackboard chalk as the alternative source. On the contrary, Nature is generous with her calcium—it's in so many foods that we find it hard to understand how the dairy council managed to claim such a monopoly. **Beans, nuts, greens (the darker and leafier, the better), grains, sea vegetables, sesame seeds (and tahini, or sesame butter), salmon and sardines with bones, soup made with animal bones (and a tablespoon of wine vinegar to leach out the bone calcium), and unsulphured blackstrap molasses** all abound in this essential mineral.

Instead of obsessing on ways to infuse calcium, take care not to lose it. Animal protein sources, concentrated sugars, alcohol, and nicotine all have been shown to affect calcium levels deleteriously. Adding dairy products to your diet as a way of compensating for lost calcium is a catch-22. While dairy products are high in calcium, they are also high in animal proteins—which ultimately leach the calcium from your body. Limiting or avoiding these foods or substances should be your first defense against calcium deficiency diseases.

MINERALS, WATER, AND MINERAL WATERS

Because calcium is the obsession *du jour*, too many of us have lost sight of the fact that it's one of dozens of minerals crucial to human life. All electrolytic action—essentially, that tiny electrical current the body relies on to perform everything from thinking to flexing a bicep—relies on the presence of these inorganic substances, normally derived from diet. Yet most of us are deficient in minerals. Either they're not in our produce (because the soil is void of them) and are absent from our water (thanks to modern water treatment), or we're unable to either assimilate those we ingest (due to insufficient stomach acid, or pharmaceutical interference, or plaque-lined intestines) or keep our reserves (excessive animal protein and stress both draw down our account). Osteoporosis, bad as it is, is but one of scores of diseases that can be attributed to a mineral deficiency.

The solution, as we see it, is exactly that: a solution. Mineral water is loaded with much of what we're missing in a form we can most readily absorb. The longevity of certain peoples—most of them high-altitude dwellers, whose only water source is mountain or glacial runoff—is thought to be traceable to their mineral ingestion. Those of us who don't live in the Himalayas can nonetheless avail ourselves of bottled waters such as Perrier, Volvic, and San Pellegrino—each of which has a mineral concentration of at least 500 ppm (parts per million). Spring water is probably our second choice, but beware of what you buy: a no-name bottled water might well have come from a pipe running off a slag heap in western Pennsylvania.

We'd caution against using tap water, if only because so many undesirable inorganic materials are in it. By the time it comes through your tap it's been loaded down with phosphates (to retard the leaching of lead from old pipes or joints), fluoride, and a host of anticontaminants to kill bacteria. Well water, once thought to be pure simply because so many rural folk relied on it, is now so likely to be a fount of nitrates, heavy metals, and bacteria that it makes the distilled water you put in your iron look delectable.

THAT OTHER ESSENTIAL MINERAL

Salt is something our bodies must have. Sodium, when ionized, is an essential electrolyte, or electricity conductor. It occurs naturally in plants. The salt derived from sun-evaporated seawater is 77 percent sodium chloride, with a complement of trace minerals that aids in its utilization.

Much has been said about the relationship between our high intake of land-mined salt and hypertension, or high blood pressure. It should be noted that the foods that are notoriously high in salt also happen to be those that are high in fat, cholesterol, refined flour, refined sugar, or other denatured foods. Denatured foods require salt and fat for flavor. High blood pressure is primarily a result of the saturated fat, which accumulates and hardens in the arteries, clogging them to the point where the volume of blood passing through exerts considerable pressure on the arterial walls. Salt increases blood volume, and so may raise blood pressure. But it's at best a secondary cause.

Regulating salt intake, according to a recent Canadian study, may help only those whose blood pressure is already problematic due to arteriosclerosis.

Our advice: Cook with just enough sea salt or seaweed to bring out the natural flavor of grains and vegetables. Get rid of the salt cellar on your table.

Alternatively, one of our favorite seasonings happens also to be the most healthful. Called gomashio, or sesame salt, it's a combination of roasted sea salt and roasted sesame seeds, ground together until the oil from the seeds coats the granules of salt. You can make it yourself: Simply roast the salt in an iron or stainless steel skillet, roast the sesame the same way, combine them in a ratio of 1 part salt to 14 parts seed, and grind thoroughly in a *surabachi*, a ceramic bowl with ridges inside sold at health food stores. You can also buy it prepared.

The benefits of gomashio are at least twofold. One, the oil-coated salt won't cause thirst. Two, the oil seems to help in the transport of salt across the cellular membrane. We also think it tastes good. But as with any salt, don't overdo it: food that tastes salty is *too* salty.

WHAT'S FOR DINNER?

Dinner can be what you've always cooked, minus the meat ... or it can be an adventure in new foods, new cooking methods, and new taste sensations. There's pasta ... and then there's **spinach fettucini with artichoke hearts, olives and sun-dried tomatoes, or jerusalem artichoke angel hair with steamed broccoli, cauliflower, and carrots in a tofu sesame saute.**

There's rice 'n beans ... and then there's **brown rice with adzuki beans, hijiki seaweed, and a saute of yellow squash, zucchini, and onion, seasoned with gomashio.**

There's soup and salad ... and then there's **miso-kombu soup and a taboule salad with tomatoes, lemon juice, and bean sprouts on hearts of romaine.**

There's meat and potatoes ... and then there's **baked lemon garlic filet of sole with brown rice and baked butternut squash.**

There's burger and fries . . . and then there's **veggie or tofu burger and a baked potato seasoned with gomashio and chives, along with a salad of red leaf lettuce, red pepper, tomatoes, and sauteed shitake mushrooms**.

The possibilities are endless (see our "Getting It All Together" chapter for more ideas). It's simply that most of us have acquired a repertoire that revolves around meat, and so our minds go dead when it comes to imagining meals without it. That, and we're not sure how to incorporate things like tofu, how to make sauces without butter and flour, or how to season with seaweed and tamari instead of table salt.

Our suggestion: get some decent cookbooks on the subject. You'll get new ideas, and you'll learn all those little tricks that can transform an off-putting food into an appetizing one. Tofu, for example, can look like clots of soured milk in a stir-fry if not pressed beforehand to extract excess fluid. And it can taste pretty bland if not marinated in, say, lemon zest and rice wine. We've made it easy for you to get started on this new adventure by listing our favorite cookbooks at the back of this book. Every day, it seems, another renowned chef produces a volume of low-fat, high-flavor, mostly vegetarian recipes that showcase all the foods we've mentioned. (See the Appendix for some of our favorites.)

As you experiment with different recipes, bear in mind that some cooking methods are preferable to others, not only because they make the most of taste but also because they keep nutrients intact and digestion optimal. Some diets stress the need for "raw" everything; others, including the diet billions of Chinese have adhered to for centuries, advocate cooking virtually everything, albeit lightly. We embrace these extremes by suggesting you eat foods prepared in a variety of ways—for balance and to avoid monotony. Weight loss research shows that the enzymes retained in uncooked foods aid in their metabolization and may effectively "burn" harder-to-digest foods that otherwise putrefy or get stored as fat.

In general, **if you "eat with the seasons"—fresh fruits and raw, blanched, chilled, or grilled fresh vegetables in the summer; lightly steamed, stir-fried, stewed, or baked root vegetables and dried fruits in the winter—you'll nurture body and soul.** Stir-frying or sauteeing is always preferable to frying or deep frying; light steaming is always preferable to boiling in water, as most of the vitamins and minerals get drained off with the water. Stewing is something else again: the juices or essences are retained as part of the end product, be it soup or fruit. Crockpots accomplish this beautifully, particularly since they rely on low heat: high heat, or prolonged cooking, destroys the nutritional value of many foods. Beware of microwaves: they're best for reheating, not cooking, as they change food's molecular structure so quickly that it's hard to prevent enzyme destruction.

Even if you're not floundering in the kitchen, consider taking a cooking class: vegetarian, low-fat, or Asian. Learning a new cuisine is an excellent way to stop obsessing about what you *shouldn't have* and start rejoicing in all the new and tasty foods that await you. When you're eating for wellness, you dwell on what you're *eating*; when you're eating for weight loss, you dwell on what you're *not* eating.

Janet, 43, a Feeling Light seminar participant, came to us programmed with a lifetime of cultural biases that made our menu suggestions look like they were from Mars. Prior to joining us, Janet had been cooking a "United Nations" array of dishes, from tacos and sushi to beef bourgignon, from lobster Newburgh and coquilles

St. Jacques to kielbasa and pierogi. Her husband's Polish background, her German background, and a stint in Ladies' Home Journal's food department had made her quite a cook—and quite a pastry chef.

"I was always the person asked to bring dessert," laughs Janet. "One of my trademark dishes was this pie with a chocolate graham-cracker crust, a layer of cheesecake and sour cream, a layer of brittle chocolate, chocolate mousse, and chocolate whipped cream on top!"

These days, says Janet, a former chronic bronchitis sufferer, four or five days will pass without a single dinner entree of meat, "and my husband doesn't even notice it's gone. We'll have pasta with fresh vegetables, salad with a platter of raw vegetables and hummus, highly seasoned Spanish rice with vegetables, chilies stuffed with buckwheat groats and vegetables. We haven't lost any of the spice," she notes, "but we sure have cut way back on the meat, dairy, and fat." When she goes out for lunch, Janet chooses an Indian restaurant because its buffet is laden with spicy vegetarian dishes. How can a girl who grew up equating comfort with a chocolate egg cream have reprogrammed her eating, cooking, and dining out habits?

"It hasn't been painless," she admits. "I've tried making an egg cream out of soy milk and seltzer, and it just isn't the same.

"But you know, I really enjoy the good choices I make as much as the bad choices I used to make. I've learned to enjoy a new group of things, not because they're substitutes, but because they're part of a different life I like. Now, when I'm out of broccoli or the piece I have isn't fresh, I really miss it! Who would have thought that was possible? Certainly not me!"

Eliminating foods in your diet is admittedly a drag; adding them shouldn't be. Try new things! Focus on the dazzling array of choices in nature's bounty, and you won't waste a moment lamenting the loss of colorings, dyes, hydrogenated fats, saturated fats, preservatives, high fructose corn syrup, olestra, nitrites, or other poisons we've discussed.

EATING OUT

Restaurants couldn't care less about your health—unless they can profit by caring. They're in the business of making food tasty and/or abundant, because the more you enjoy the food they prepare, the more you'll pay for it, and the more you'll keep coming back for it.

And yet, our clients don't ask, "*Can* I eat at a restaurant?" They ask, "*What* can I eat at a restaurant?"

Eating out is our culture, after all. The demands of work and family push meal preparation out of the picture. We buy our breakfast off a truck, eat our lunches out of a deli wrapper, and pick up dinner not from a market but from a take-out kitchen. Dining out as an occasional social pleasure has evolved into a regular business expense, where even breakfast carries an agenda. For a fact, there's no getting out of eating out.

Fortunately, more restaurants are finding it profitable to court your healthier instincts. Health as the foremost concern on the menu is reflected in the proliferation of so-called California cuisine, wherein even the lowly pizza is elevated to health food status with freshly prepared sauce, roasted vegetables, and seasonings from Italy to Indonesia. Increasingly, short-order cooks who've never seen a fresh pepper cross their chopping block are willing to accommodate requests for no-salt, no-grease, or no-sauce preparations. The sheer numbers of weight-conscious patrons have forced the industry to acknowledge that what the customer wants is no longer pure indulgence.

Still, bastions of beef 'n butter abound. For many who

work in office parks or along shopping strips, there's Red
Lobster, Sizzler, or McDonald's to choose from for lunch
outings, where health is supposedly a salad bar groaning
with buckets of blue cheese dressing, Bac-Os, and Jello-ed
fruit. Getting a quick bite to eat at any hour still means
dropping in at a diner or a TGIF, whose encyclopedic
menus offer precious little that hasn't been deep-fried,
griddle-pressed, boiled beyond recognition, ladled with
lard, or scooped right out of an industrial-size can. Aside
from an unadorned baked potato, a poached egg, or a half
grapefruit, we can't think of an item there we'd endorse.
At fast-food franchises, there's even less.

We can offer you several survival strategies. Avoid franchises altogether, unless it's a franchise like California
Kitchen. Standardized food shipments, cooks trained by
rote, and an aspiration for sameness give these places
precious little flexibility to accommodate individual requests. If you find yourself at a salad bar, bear in mind
that **spinach** leaves are preferable to iceberg lettuce, **fresh
veggies** are better than mushrooms from a can, **kidney
beans** are way better than cottage cheese, and **vinaigrette
or oil 'n' vinegar** is a no-contest winner over any of the
salad dressings.
 Choose restaurants where fresh or vegetarian are terms
practiced, not just preached. **Middle Eastern and Far Eastern cuisines—Moroccan, Pakistani, Indian, Vietnamese,
Japanese, or Chinese—as well as some Mediterranean
(Greek, Turkish, or Italian) are usually good bets.** Select
fish or vegetable entrees where you can specify **steaming,
poaching, stir-frying, stewing, or grilling** methods of
preparation. Bear in mind that you're dining out primarily
for the social exchange, which won't be at all affected by
what you order.
 Or go ahead and order the filet mignon with shoestring

potatoes and Caesar salad. Once in a while—once every month or so—we encourage you to treat yourself. There's no harm in occasional splurges. It's the cumulative effect of three meals a day, day in and day out, over years and decades, that does the real damage. If giving into seduction now and then allows you to keep your body an unviolated temple for most of the month, then we're all for it.

ALCOHOL

The Chinese have argued for centuries that a little alcohol, especially during winter, is good for balance. Alcohol's hot, acrid nature quickens the flow of blood and the flow of chi. More recent science shows that consumption of **red wine** can actually lessen the risk of heart disease by lowering cholesterol. Most cultures have long regarded wine as a valuable digestive, particularly when helping the body break down saturated fats and animal protein.

We're neither for nor against alcohol. Our position is consistently one of moderation, unless you are immoderately ill. If you're basically healthy—albeit over- or underweight—we see no reason why you shouldn't enjoy a glass of wine with dinner once every two weeks or so. Choose a California wine, as they're less likely to contain sulfites, or a wine labeled "organic" or "sulfite-free."

Beer is more of a mixed bag: on the one hand, a **dark porter or stout** is full of the vitamin B complex; on the other, many dark-looking beers are devoid of vitamins and full of sugar and chemicals. Despite the fact that beer is made from fermented grains like barley and hops, inferior ingredients and overprocessing typically render the brew second-best. Imports and microbrewed ales and stouts may be your best bet. Still, unless your objective is weight gain, an "occasional" beer means once a month: As any beer drinker can attest, beer is expanding.

Refined alcohol such as **vodka, gin, or scotch** should be limited to those rare special occasions—50th wedding anniversaries, your 40th birthday—where you're indulging just to remind yourself of what you're not missing. Avoid altogether sugary, creamy, or syrupy concoctions such as daiquiris, brandy alexanders, sours, mai tais, and the like.

CHEATING

"Can I eat pizza?"

"You mean no ice cream, ever again?"

"What about the holidays?"

"What happens if I cheat?"

If you've ever dieted, then you know as surely as you breathe that you're going to cheat, sooner or later. That's because dieting is deprivation and discipline. Success is achieved by what you cut out and measured by what you've lost. Because dieting never improves diet, failure is an inevitability—it's only a matter of degree.

But Feeling Light is not a diet. We don't want to see you starve yourself, or stick to some insane regimen of excruciatingly boring foods. We're advising you to change what you eat, not stop eating. Every healthful food you ingest, every healthful eating habit you adopt—you come out ahead. You can't fail; you can only do better and better.

Say you cut out the beef and beef up on the whole grains, but pretty much draw the line there. Or maybe you substitute fish for meat, rice milk for cow's milk, and honey for sugar. Or maybe you just cut out all processed foods. Those are good choices, never mind what others you may make. You're that much closer to achieving balance.

But here's what we've observed: every little step you take toward balance makes you feel that much more empowered to take the next step. You feel better; you look better. That's what makes our clients keep coming to Feeling Light. They can see and feel what's happening as a result of every little modification they make. Their skin clears up. Their hair shines. Their nails are strong. They sleep better. Their disposition improves. Yeast infections stop plaguing them. Allergies lessen, asthma eases, bronchitis disappears. They feel lighter—and in most cases, they *are* lighter.

And as they approach a balance of mind, body, and soul, they feel fewer of the cravings they felt certain would derail them in their mission. They acquire a wholly new set of palate pleasers. Just as in physics, the closer one gets to balance, the easier it becomes to achieve—and the easier it is to maintain.

Of course, even the most resolute of our participants experience lapses, periods where old habits reclaim territory they'd lost to healthful habits. This isn't cheating; this is normal human behavior. One of our clients was on the verge of ditching Feeling Light simply because she'd "regressed," as though the program wouldn't work if she didn't adopt it lock, stock, and barrel. Nonsense! We're not absolutists. Moderation is our watchword, because balance can never be achieved by extreme measures. The beauty of acquiring healthful eating habits is that every one counts in your favor, but none that you let drop count against you. **If you drop a piece of the picture we've assembled for you here, there's always a new day, a cleansing fast, and a clean slate with which to begin anew.** Cheating is not possible. There are simply good choices, better choices, and optimal choices awaiting you.

CHAPTER SEVEN

Super Nutrition

Immunity, Vitality, and Weight Management through Supplementation

"*I don't see how I can stick with this program. I feel hungry* all the time. *I have these cravings. Especially for sweets.*"

Cravings? *Of course you have cravings. Your body is crying out for the nutrients it lacks!*

That's right. In this country, even people severely overweight are nonetheless starving—starving for essential amino acids, enzymes, trace minerals, and organic chemicals fundamental to physical and mental function that are all normally derived from food and water. The only way the body knows how to get what it needs is to eat, and

the forces it employs—hunger and cravings—are irresis-
tible. Our nutritionally deficient clients truly "hunger" for
food, despite the fact that they've just eaten. It's not fuel
they need; their gasoline gauge reads full. But because
their vitamin and mineral gauges remain in the red zone,
that gnawing, needy, demanding voice whines, "I want
something."

More often than not, that voice gets answered with
cookies, candy, ice cream, chips, munchies—whatever
holds the promise of quick and easy gratification. One bite,
one chip never seems to satisfy. And yet, even after the
bag or carton is empty, the voice nags: "I want something
else."

The entire diet industry would have you believe that
successful weight loss depends on tuning out this voice.
You're to stifle your urges or discipline yourself to disre-
gard them. As if you could! Cravings are not easily ignored
because they're not meant to be: they're your body's way
of alerting you to a deficiency, one that must be corrected
if energy, immunity, and physical and mental acuity are
to be maintained.

Alas, a craving is rarely articulate about what *exactly* is
wanting, so we ingest what's nearest and most appetizing—sugar, salt, fat—and in so doing we aggravate the
deficiency. As we've discussed already, refined flour, refined sugar, hydrogenated fats, and land-mined salt draw
down the body's reserves of vitamins and minerals because these foods have been stripped of the nutritional
packaging Nature intended for their digestion. Without
their own complement of vitamins and minerals, they have
to "borrow" from *your* nutritional stores in order to be
assimilated. These foods, in effect, are not only "empty"
calories but also *thieving* ones. Hence binging on barren
nourishment virtually guarantees that cravings will return

with a vengeance. Cravings are at the root of the vicious cycle that keeps dieters dieting . . . and failing.

We believe in listening to the body—listening carefully, and taking the time to figure out what's instigating these cravings rather than just smother the voice with a bag of potato chips. We have seen in countless instances how cravings can be quieted simply by administering the nutrients denied our clients by their diet of denatured foods. The results are often dramatic. We've seen lifelong chocoholics kick the habit by supplementing with magnesium. We've seen incurable sweet tooths "cured" of their craving by upping their intake of chromium.

And we've helped Feeling Light participants who've insisted they're too tired, too draggy, too depressed, or too overwhelmed to change their eating habits to get with the program—simply by giving them the energy-boosting vitamins and "superfoods" that empower them to change. Supplements, in short, can jump-start a successful eating program by answering the nutritional needs that otherwise derail the most dedicated dieter.

Supplements can also dramatically alter your appearance. Your skin, your hair, your nails—all benefit visibly, where no lotion or "overnight" creme ever had the slightest effect.

"People keep asking me if I've had a face-lift," laughs Mary Jo, 57, a client of ours who's been supplementing for relief from allergies. "And it's true, my skin is much firmer, shinier, more elastic. That puffiness under my eyes is gone."

Even where other aging influences are at work, supplements can help check the damage. Smoking, for example, exerts a terrific drain on the body's mineral reserves, inhibits vitamin absorption, and impairs immunity; the optimal solution, of course, is to quit. But for people who won't quit, supplements are all the more vital.

> *Lifelong smoker Marilyn, at 70, says that while her friends are going to the doctor with all manner of complaints ("looking old and acting old"), she's tearing up the dance floor. "When my daughter introduces me to her friends and tells them my age, they all figure I had plastic surgery," she notes. "Then when I tell them I'm on a complete set of vitamins, they all get out pencil and paper. They want to take what I'm taking."*

BUT WHAT ABOUT DIET?

Even those of us eating right—choosing whole grains and organically grown produce, minimizing meat and dairy, and limiting sweets and alcohol—can benefit from supplementation. Not everything we eat is as nutritionally complete as it could be, because few of us are growing our own produce and eating it ripe from the garden. The "fresh" produce we buy may well have been picked green, shipped hard, gassed to ripen, and refrigerated to extend its shelf life—all factors known to compromise nutritional value. Organic fruits and vegetables have arguably a more complete complement of nutrients, but not all the produce we eat is organic. Nor is every meal we consume free of butter, salt, or sugar, especially when we dine out. Factors completely beyond our control, such as pollution or stress, continue to draw on our nutritional reserves. And there were years where we made little or no deposits to our savings, eating the wrong foods or not enough of the right foods.

Hence, to stay solvent, we supplement. We eat as

healthfully as we can, and then we add vitamins, minerals, enzymes, and fiber extracted from natural sources as "insurance" against bounced-check charges. To paraphrase Dr. Joel Wallach, the Nobel Prize nominee who decries our nation's mineral insolvency, which would you rather pay for: $70,000 for hip replacement surgery or a dime a day for extra calcium? As insurance policies go, supplementation turns out to be mighty cheap. And as prevention programs go, there's simply no better way, in our experience, to keep the doctors away.

Don't be fooled by a "one-a-day" multivitamin! Wallach estimates that there are some sixteen vitamins and sixty minerals the human body needs to function optimally and fend off degenerative disease. Even if he's only partially right, it's clear that the multivitamin you swallow as your current insurance plan is not up to the job. If it were, it'd have to be the size of a door. The reason you can swallow it is that vitamin manufacturers use as dosage guidelines the RDA, or recommended daily allowances—amounts adequate to sustain life, but not to protect against the ravages of modern life. Recent research on the role of antioxidants in preventing cancer and slowing down the aging process suggests that the RDA is woefully out of date. Selenium, to cite but one mineral, is widely acknowledged to be among the most potent of antioxidants, but it has yet to elicit any guidelines from the FDA regarding proper dosage.

That's why you see some people popping handfuls of pills: they'd rather be safe than sorry. Yet most of our clients, understandably, resist the idea of making every meal a vitamin ordeal. So we've come up with a more streamlined, user-friendly approach. We call it:

—THE FEELING LIGHT SMOOTHIE—

It's a blender drink. It's breakfast. It's a total infusion of essential vitamins, minerals, EFAs, protein, and fiber. And our clients simply love it.

> *"It perks me right up. It puts me in a good mood. And let me tell you, it's an extraordinary thing for me to give up solid food and drink this thick green stuff!"*
> *—Madelyne, 45, mother and singer*

> *"I'd been suffering from low energy ever since my daughter was born until I started drinking the Smoothie. It charges me up for the day. I drink half in the morning, half in the afternoon, and I don't get those three-o'clock-slumps anymore. And the baby loves it: She asks for 'the green juice!'"*
> *—Marianne, 32-year-old mother of a toddler*

> *"I can't start my day without it. It makes me feel so healthy, so energetic, I feel like I can make healthier choices the rest of the day."*
> *—Debbie, occupational therapist*

The Smoothie consists of the following ingredients—but be creative! Experiment with different proportions of fruits and juices, or try freezing the banana and strawberries to make a thicker, colder concoction. You don't have to follow this recipe to the letter; the important thing is that you tailor it to your own tastes.

Blend well in a blender:

1 cup rice milk, soy milk, apple juice, orange
  juice, or other fruit juice
1 whole ripe banana
4 fresh strawberries
1 teaspoon blackstrap molasses
1 tablespoon aloe vera juice
1 tablespoon black cherry juice concentrate
1 tablespoon powdered "green" formulation
1 to 2 tablespoons powdered brewer's or nutritional yeast
1 teaspoon raw, organic bee pollen—loose, not
  in tablets or capsules
1 tablespoon flaxseed oil, or a combination of
  flaxseed and other oils high in EFAs, such as
  borage, sunflower, sesame, and pumpkin.

Some of these ingredients will no doubt mystify you; let
us demystify them.

- **Blackstrap molasses**, the unrefined distillation of sugarcane, is loaded with the minerals that we refine out
  of white sugar. It's high in calcium, potassium, and
  iron.
- **Aloe vera juice** is an herbal extract that soothes,
  cleanses, and tonifies the gastrointestinal tract. It can
  be used to heal ulcers and relieve colitis and diverti-
  culitus. It's particularly effective in detoxifying the intestines.
- **Black cherry juice** is a blood purifier high in vitamin
  C. Like strawberries, this fruit aids in the dissolution
  and neutralization of uric acid, which can lead to gout
  and kidney stones. It also tastes great!

- **Green formulations** typically contain chlorophyll, one of the best blood purifiers, blood oxygenators, and blood builders found in nature; it can be used to treat anemia. Wheat grass, barley grass, alfalfa, chlorella, and **spirulina,** one of the blue-green algaes (a "superfood" we shall discuss), are the primary sources of "green" in most formulations. Good formulations also include lecithin and herbs such as licorice root, kelp, red clover, ginkgo, and gotu-kolu. (See our chapter on herbs.)
- **Brewer's yeast,** also known as nutritional yeast, is made from hops. It contains all the B vitamins, sixteen amino acids, key minerals such as phosphorus and chromium, and protein. For boosting immunity, for energy, and for endurance, there are few supplements that can compare to brewer's yeast.
- **Bee pollen** is the powdery yellow substance bees collect from flower stamens. If we were to be shipwrecked on a desert island for months, this is the supplement we'd hope we'd have for the duration: it's a whole food. All the B vitamins, vitamin C, EFAs, key enzymes, seven minerals, carotene, and protein are present in high concentrations. It's a surefire source of energy, especially for those three o'clock doldrums.
- **Flaxseed oil** is a prime source of essential fatty acids (EFAs), chiefly linoleic acid, which we literally cannot live without. All too many Americans are deficient in EFAs, as we pointed out earlier, and in the campaign to eliminate all fats from the diet, too many good sources of EFAs are being thrown out with the saturated fat bathwater. We've seen so-called compulsive eaters cured of cravings simply by boosting their EFA levels with flaxseed oil. It also serves as a source of magnesium, potassium, B vitamins, protein, and zinc.
- **Borage oil**, another superunsaturated fat source, is

rich in GLAs, essential fatty acids that are particularly helpful in treating PMS (**evening primrose oil** is also highly effective, but a lot more expensive). Polyunsaturated oils derived from sunflower, sesame and pumpkin also help correct EFA deficiency. Supplement with 1,000 mg of one or a combination of these oils once a day.

Once you try our Smoothie, you'll see—feel!—why our clients swear by it and why we lovingly call it "rocket fuel." It is highly effective, not merely because it combines everything you may be currently lacking, but because it conveys these supplements in their most assimilable form. The more "whole" the food—meaning the more closely the supplement resembles the natural source from which it was derived—the more readily your body recognizes, absorbs, and utilizes its nutritional constituents.

Supplements are *not* created equal: "Foods" like spirulina are best, liquids and powders are very good, capsules are fine, tablets are acceptable, and natural is always preferable to anything synthetically produced or augmented with artificial colorings, preservatives, sweeteners, starches, or fillers. Read the label very carefully. For example, D-Alpha Tocopherol is the form of vitamin E we recommend, and yet its synthetic counterpart—an inferior product—goes by Dl-Alpha Tocopherol. A health food store or mail-order house whose stock is reputably all-natural will offer each vitamin and mineral in a variety of forms—liquid, powder, capsule, tablet, etc. The less foodlike the form, the more important it is to consume the supplement with a meal, because then your stomach will then receive it in more or less the nutritional "package" of proteins and lipids your body can assimilate. For maximal effect, supplements should be taken over the course of a day, rather than all at once in the morning.

TISSUE CLEANSING

All-around nutritious as the Smoothie is, its curative powers will be compromised if your gastrointestinal tract is lined with years of residue, which blocks absorption and keeps toxifying your lymphatic system. For this very reason, the various cleansing and detoxification programs we've already discussed play a critical role in the success of the Feeling Light program.

If, however, you're not ready to engage in a cleansing fast—or if you've fasted and want to maintain "a clean slate"—the following bulk additives will help your stomach and intestines work at peak efficiency. That is, food will be "burned" clean, and indigestible waste will spend very little time in transit out of the body. Most importantly, residues from years of non-clean burning foods—animal proteins, saturated fats, dairy by-products—will be dislodged, along with the harmful bacteria that inhabit them. A host of colonic disorders, such as colitis, diverticulitis, and even cancer may be prevented by restoring and maintaining bowel health. Dietary fibers are not to be confused with laxatives, which are bowel stimulants that can wreak havoc with intestinal balance to the point where bowel movement is virtually impossible without them.

- **Flaxmeal**—Ground flax seed is a natural fiber that offers the "brooming" action of nondigestible cellulose, the soothing properties of soluble fiber, the antibacterial, fungal, and viral protection of lignins, and the nutrition of EFAs, boron, and potassium. Its combination of fibers has been shown to scrape carcinogenic substances from the colon wall while protecting the mucous lining, which safeguards against digestive juices and invasive bacteria. The woody substances called lignins lower cholesterol and, when mixed with beneficial bacteria in the colon, form antioxidant compounds thought to protect against breast cancer.

Recommended dosage: Start with a half teaspoon mixed in eight to twelve ounces of water or juice, and build up to one to two tablespoons in water or juice, followed by another glass or two, daily. The more liquid you use it with, the better it works.

- **Psyllium seed husk**—This nonnutritive fiber is often prescribed as a stool softener, but we find it an effective colon cleanser and healer. As a mucilage, psyllium is also invaluable for picking up fats off the colon wall and helping regulate blood sugar levels. It may also be helpful in curbing appetite, because when mixed with water or juice, it swells into a bulky mass quickly. Metamucil and Citrical are synthetic preparations containing psyllium; we prefer unprocessed, natural husks.

  Recommended dosage: Start with a half teaspoon mixed in eight to twelve ounces of water or juice, and build up to one to two tablespoons in water or juice, followed by another glass or two, daily. Again, the more liquid you drink, the more effective it will be. Psyllium may be mixed with flaxmeal.

- **Triphala**—From India comes this bowel cleanser and fat eliminator, a combination of three fruits (amla, behada, and harada) also used in lowering cholesterol, detoxifying the blood and liver, increasing red blood cells and hemoglobin, and tonifying the entire digestive tract. Daily use helps promote the absorption of B vitamins. High in Vitamin C, this laxative may also boost immunity. Triphala may be taken with psyllium and flaxmeal simultaneously.

  Recommended dosage: Two tablets three times daily.

- **Lactobacillus bifidus and acidophilus**—If you've ever
  been on an antibiotic, or if you suffer from gas, diarrhea, or intestinal cramping, you're probably woefully
  deficient in "friendly" bacteria. Lactobacteria normally
  inhabit the intestines and help in digestion and healthy
  bowel action, but they can be wiped out by poor eating
  habits or medication. A diet heavy in hard-to-digest
  animal protein will kill them off, since undigested protein will putrefy in the intestines and welcome "bad"
  bacteria that compete with the good. To reestablish lac-
  tobacterial populations, supplement with granules or
  capsules; live-culture yogurt has nowhere near enough
  bacteria to replace what's been lost, and many people
  cannot tolerate the lactose, or milk sugar, on which the
  bacteria feed.

  Recommended dosage: Start with two capsules three
  times a day for one month. Cut down to one capsule
  three times a day the following month; then to one
  capsule two times a day. If you've been on antibiotics,
  or have suffered a chronic bowel condition, reestablish-
  ing lactobacteria may take longer. As a liquid, lacto-
  bacterial supplement can be added to the Smoothie.

FAT FIGHTERS

Once intestinal health is restored, wellness and weight
management can go hand in hand. The key is to boost
metabolism, either by stimulating the thyroid, which is the
glandular seat of metabolic activity, or by stimulating the
digestive process, typically with enzymes that break down
fats. Other substances then help carry unwanted cholesterol and lipids out of the body.

The following thyroid activators, enzymes, and amino
acids comprise supplementation you may take until
weight is no longer an issue.

- **Coenzyme Q10, or "CoQ10"**—Preliminary research shows that this substance—a powerful antioxidant that resembles vitamin E in molecular structure—may help people lose weight by restoring their ability to burn food, particularly fats. The fact that nearly half of the overweight subjects studied for this enzyme were deficient in it suggests that CoQ10 plays a vital role in "firing up" the metabolic furnace. In addition, it boosts the immune system, is thought to prevent and control cancer, and may reduce high blood pressure and heart disease. Because its presence in human tissue declines naturally with age, supplementation is recommended even where weight is not a problem.
Recommended dosage: 30 mg at breakfast and again at dinner.

- **Chromium Picolinate**—An estimated 9 out of 10 Americans are chromium deficient, which may well explain why 1 out of every 3 is overweight: Chromium stabilizes blood sugar levels by ensuring that insulin is used properly. Erratic blood sugar levels can account for the "hungry all the time" feeling many of our clients complain of, despite the fact that they're eating constantly. A chromium deficiency translates into the sort of nonspecific craving for food true hypoglycemics feel: a blood sugar "low" that spurs binges on quick-fix foods high in sugar and fat. These foods, in turn, spike blood sugar without supplying the chromium necessary to prevent the ensuing "crash."
Recommended dosage: 100 mcg at breakfast and again at dinner.

- **Kelp**—While it's a seaweed, kelp is not often eaten as a food. Used in its granulated or powdered form, it can stand in as a salt substitute, seasoning, or condi-

ment. But because of its concentration of vitamins and minerals, kelp is most commonly ingested in tablet form as a supplement. High in iodine, this seaweed stimulates the thyroid to release thyroxin, the hormone responsible for raising metabolism.
Recommended dosage: One or two tablets with each meal.

• **Spirulina**—In addition to bee pollen, we'd sure hope to find this blue-green algae in our knapsacks on that desert island. It offers an extreme concentration of protein, essential fatty acids, B12, iron, essential amino acids, chlorophyll, and a blue pigment that is thought to boost the immune system. Because its protein content helps stabilize blood sugar, it curbs appetite by balancing out the highs and lows that provoke eating binges. As a metabolic activator, this algae speeds weight loss by firing up the furnace. Spirulina also helps in fasting, providing perfect nutrition and energy while helping cleanse the body of toxins.
Recommended dosage: One-half to one scoop of the powder once daily; in pill form, one to two tablets, three times a day.

• **Lecithin**—We can't think of anyone who wouldn't benefit from this essential fatty substance—a lifesaving fat solvent. Cell membranes are composed of it. So are the meninges, the tissues protecting the brain. Lecithin helps us absorb thiamine and vitamin A, promotes brain function, and boosts energy. For those who are at risk for heart disease, lecithin is vital for its role as an emulsifier, protecting arteries and organs from fatty deposits, which build up into hard plaques. Because lecithin aids in the digestion of fat and makes cholesterol and other lipids water-soluble, it's an effective tool in weight management.

Recommended dosage: Two tablespoons of granulated lecithin, on food or cereal or in a Smoothie, daily.

- **L-Carnitine**—This amino acid is thought to aid weight loss by revving up metabolism and converting stored body fat into energy. It helps control hypoglycemia, and is known to prevent fatty buildup in the arteries and tissues. It also boosts the antioxidant properties of vitamins C and E.
  Recommended dosage: One 250 mg to 500 mg tablet at breakfast and again at dinner.

INVESTING IN LONG-TERM HEALTH

No chapter on supplements would be complete without a discussion of antioxidants—substances that slow the aging process by gobbling up unstable, free-roaming, destructive molecules called free radicals. Antioxidants have received quite a bit of press for their role in preventing cancer; there isn't a multivitamin supplement on the shelves that doesn't now proclaim the virtues of its vitamin A, C, and E quotient. In fact, we tell our clients to keep up their PACES, meaning they supplement with the proven cancer-fighters: pycnogenol, vitamin A (beta-carotene), vitamin C, vitamin E, and selenium. To this arsenal we might well add the potent antioxidant coenzyme Q10, discussed above.

- **Pycnogenol**—This supplement is among the newest in the arsenal of antioxidants. Derived from both grape seeds and pine bark, pycnogenol is almost exclusively found in supplemental form.
  Recommended dosage: 30 mg at breakfast and dinner.

- **Vitamin A**—If you've read about the importance of beta-carotene, then you know how Vitamin A has been shown to ward off colds and flu, repair damaged epithelial (skin) tissue, heal ulcers, destroy carcinogens, shield against pollution (which depresses immune function), and generally retard the effects of continual bodily wear and tear.
  Recommended dosage: 10,000 iu twice daily, with breakfast and dinner.

- **Vitamin C**—Even the most nutritionally cheated American knows the importance of getting enough of this immunity-boosting vitamin, which has been used (in adequate dosages) to prevent everything from the common cold to cancer. It repairs damaged tissue, protects against blood clotting and bruising, helps heal wounds, and boosts output of antistress hormones.
  Recommended dosage: In esterified form (such as Ester-C), 2,000 to 3,000 mg is sufficient. Take 1,000 mg with each meal.

- **Vitamin E**—This powerful antioxidant is most recognized for its visible effect on hair, nails, and skin. Taken in concert with vitamin C, it offers more than double the protection against cancer and other degenerative diseases caused by inadequate immune function.
  Recommended dosage: We recommend D-Alpha Tocopherol. For people under 40, 400 iu daily is best; for those over 40, 400 iu twice daily.

- **Selenium**—Like vitamin C, this trace element revs up the body's defenses to fight against infection. As an antioxidant, it works best in concert with vitamin E. Its role in maintaining tissue elasticity makes it useful in preventing heart disease.

Recommended dosage: 50 mcg at both breakfast and dinner.

- **Zinc Picolinate**—While zinc itself is not an antioxidant, an insuffiency of this mineral decreases the concentrations of vitamin E in the blood. Zinc is also responsible for boosting immunity, protecting the liver from damage, and ensuring reproductive health—especially prostate function. A loss of taste and smell can indicate a zinc deficiency.
  Recommended dosage: 50 mg at breakfast and again at dinner. Do not exceed 100 mg daily.

MAXIMAL WELLNESS, MINIMAL WEIGHT

For many of the individuals we've seen over the years, supplementation has been the single most important factor in reversing the downward spiral of malnutrition and obesity. Simply adjusting the balance of intestinal flora has relieved many of our clients' more chronic ailments—everything from gas and constipation to vaginitis and yeast infections. Others, unable to move off a weight "plateau" despite the most stringent of diets, have found relief from both fat and fatigue as soon as they started correcting the chemistry responsible for metabolic activity. Still others report feeling just an overall sense of health and well-being, because for the first time, their eating habits are no longer derailed by out-of-control cravings. And not only do they feel better, but they also *look* better. They can see the improvement in their skin and hair, and so can everyone else.

Like everything else we've discussed, however, supplementation works best when it's administered holistically. Nutrition is accomplished through balance; vitamins and minerals, when taken in balance, work synergistically—that is, the whole effect is much greater than the sum of its individual parts. Taking too much of one supplement while taking too little or none at all of another can disrupt this synergy. For example, vitamin E works best in the presence of adequate zinc, but an excess of zinc can cause a depletion of copper. While the guidelines we've given you here are generally appropriate, we would urge you to consult a health professional or nutritional counselor so that he or she might customize a supplementation plan for you, taking into account individual factors like size and weight, existing medical conditions, and diet.

Supplementation can help you achieve wellness, and wellness, as we can't stress enough, is the secret to weight loss. But there's much, much more to be gained by bolstering dietary nutrition.

"I haven't had a cold in four years," says Marilyn. "My OB says I'm a phenomenon, and that's after six children. Not only that: I weigh just a few pounds more than I did when I got married, and my blood pressure has gone down *since I started taking all these things."*

"I tell all my friends," she adds, "Start taking vitamins to keep yourself healthy and young and you'll find that you won't be running to the doctor all the time!"'

CHAPTER EIGHT

The Herbal Arsenal

A Prescription for Weight Management and Well-Being

Let's explore a dieting myth held dear since the invention of the girdle: *If you'd just eat less, you'd lose weight.*

It sounds logical enough, but in actual practice, it doesn't work. You eat less, you lose a few pounds, and then you hit that dreaded plateau where nothing happens despite the fact that you're eating a fraction of what you used to eat. Meals are a torment. You feel hungry, deprived, and—with so little to show for your efforts—despairing. You go back to former eating habits. The weight you lost, plus a few pounds, returns. The hell with it, you say.

Losing weight is a matter of either burning food better or eliminating it more efficiently. Because poor-quality food—white flour, white sugar, white salt, and saturated fat—doesn't burn clean, thereby leaving toxic residue that dampens metabolism and impairs elimination, it'll make you put on weight or foil your efforts to lose it. If, on the other hand, you detoxify (see our chapter on detoxification) and then consume combustible foods such as whole grains, legumes, fruits, and vegetables, then you'll burn calories and process waste more efficiently. Weight management, then, is really a matter of *waste* management.

That's where herbs enter the picture. **They can help you clear out toxins** and repair the organs suffering from years of abuse. **They can help stoke digestive fire and rev up your metabolism**. Most importantly, they can help keep your digestive and eliminative organs in tip-top shape so that every bite you eat gets maximally utilized and every bit of waste generated gets whisked out of your body.

WHY HERBS?

As we hope we've made perfectly clear by now, nothing in the human body works independently. Everything must work in concert with each other, in proper sequence. Much as internal combustion in your car requires not only spark plugs that spark but also the presence of vaporized gasoline in the valve chamber at the moment of ignition, metabolism in the human body requires that certain stomach enzymes be secreted before food can be properly utilized, that glucose is circulated to the muscles before energy can be expended, and that wastes are adequately removed and transported by the lymphatic network to the liver and kidneys for elimination.

In short, any tune-up you perform must be holistic in

nature if it's to be at all effective. You wouldn't replace your motor oil without also replacing your oil filter; likewise, it's kind of pointless to build your blood if your liver isn't toned enough to filter out blood impurities.

Herbs are ideally suited for this holistic approach because, unlike the hundreds of pharmaceuticals derived from them, herbs are multifaceted in effect and minimal in side effects. For example, consider any over-the-counter or prescription diuretic: that pill will make you lose "water weight" at the expense of vital minerals such as potassium, leaving you feeling literally drained. In contrast, the leaves and root of the herb marshmallow can be used as both a diuretic and a laxative, but all that's eliminated in the purging process are the toxins clouding your tissues. Marshmallow actually replaces minerals and vitamins—specifically vitamin A, the vitamin-B complex, calcium, zinc, iron, and iodine. The herb has been traditionally used to heal while flushing out wastes, which is of utmost importance in weight loss.

An herb is nature's medicine in its most complete form; as soon as one of its active ingredients is taken out from the whole (which is how some 60 percent of today's pharmaceuticals are made), the user is likely to experience side effects, because the mitigating or healing agents are lost in the refining process. So, given the choice between pharmaceutical derivative and natural herb, which would you choose?

THE STRATEGY

Herbs that we've found helpful in weight management are listed below, but not with the idea that you go out and buy a bottle of each. On the contrary, you're better off consulting a qualified herbalist for a regimen that's right for you, or buying a formulation that will include herbs from several of the categories we identify here. A good regimen or formula will include herbs that detoxify and rejuvenate the liver, lymph, blood, and tissues; flush out wastes; aid in circulation; promote better metabolism; suppress the appetite; and tonify your entire body to restore or maintain wellness. Many herbs straddle several categories. We've defined them here with an eye to their predominant effects in weight loss only.

Use our list as a reference, an informative guide to buying herbal formulations. Labeling laws forbid manufacturers to describe what their herbal preparations do, but with our guide in hand, you can read the list of ingredients and understand what each herb can do for you and how your body will be affected. Herbs can be taken in pill, capsule, extract, tincture, tea or whole food form; follow dosing guidelines as indicated on the package labels.

The use of herbs for weight loss is well documented in traditional literature. Take weight loss formulations until weight is no longer an issue. Use the energy-boosting herbs as needed. Herbs that aid in elimination should become a permanent feature of your daily diet.

The indications for each herb listed below have been verified by thousands of years of use by various cultures. **Be sure and avoid any preparations that include ephedra (or mahuang), guarana, damiana, or yohimbe**—stimulants that can give you heart palpitations, or worse.

The Herbs

Detoxification
- **Burdock**—Traditionally a blood purifier because of its detoxifying effects on the liver. The root cleanses toxins

from the digestive, urinary, and intestinal tracts as well. It stimulates digestion, eases indigestion, flushes out calcium deposits in the kidneys and urinary tract, promotes better kidney function, and lowers blood sugar levels. Its most active ingredient, a starch called inulin, helps in the metabolization of carbohydrates. Burdock can be purchased in Oriental markets and health food stores sliced and sauteed as a vegetable.

- **Chickweed**—Incredibly common, this weed has been known to have incredible curative powers with regard to stomach ulcers, inflamed bowels, and blood toxicity. It helps dissolve arterial plaque and fatty deposits. While used chiefly as a detoxifier, diuretic, and stomach and bowel strengthener, chickweed is also an effective appetite suppressant.

- **Dandelion**—A super liver detoxifier. This "weed" can clean out poisons accumulated from drug use, drug abuse, and excessive alcohol, boosting liver function as well as cleansing and building the blood, promoting circulation, and restoring normal gastric balance. Because the leaves are high in protein, antioxidants, vitamin B, calcium, sodium, and potassium (a mineral lost in frequent urination), dandelion is as nourishing as it is healing. Leaves are great in salad; roasted dandelion root can be simmered for an excellent coffee-like beverage.

- **Milk Thistle**—For overworked livers weakened by illness, toxicity, poor diet, or abuse, there's simply nothing better. The seeds accelerate tissue regeneration and, because they're high in antioxidants, help boost immunity to prevent further damage from infection or illness. Like chickweed, this herb has been known to prevent the buildup of plaque that causes arterial hardening and high blood pressure.

- **Oregon Grape**—Extracts of the root and rhizomes are used as an overall tonic and immunity booster. The herb is a superior blood cleanser, liver detoxifier, and infection fighter. It not only stimulates digestion but also maximizes the assimilation of vitamins and minerals. Like milk thistle, oregon grape helps cleanse the liver and so aids in weight management.

- **Pau d'Arco Bark**—Usually consumed as a tea, the capsule or extract form of this bark offers protection against viral, bacterial, and fungal infection. We recommend it as a blood purifier. It's also a blood builder.

- **Red Clover**—A blood purifier, the flower is also rich in vitamin C and the trace element selenium. It helps bolster immunity because it's a powerful antioxidant.

- **Sassafras**—Common to most any woods, sassafras acts as a detoxifier of the blood and tissues by stimulating the liver and kidneys. It eases stomach cramps and relieves water retention. Like chickweed, it's also an effective appetite suppressant. The bark of the root, which contains the active ingredients, is easily decocted into a flavorful tea, although commercial extract is also available in supermarkets.

- **Yellow Dock**—One of the best blood builders in the plant world. Its root is high in iron, vitamin A, and vitamin C. For blood, lymph, liver, or spleen disorders, there's nothing more effective. Also useful as a mild laxative and digestive aid.

Digestion and Elimination

- **Aloe**—Perhaps best known for the soothing topical applications of its gel, aloe vera juice is an effective tonic and digestive stimulant, which is why it's in our Smoothie. In capsule or powdered form, the leaves will not only relieve stubborn constipation but will also promote bile flow and better digestion.

- **Buchu**—The leaves have a healing effect on all the urinary organs by increasing urine, absorbing excessive uric acid, and relieving water retention. It's an effective treatment for bloating due to gas, and for digestive disorders.
- **Cleavers**—An overall cleansing tonic, cleavers, or goosegrass, purifies the blood and lymph chiefly through its diuretic action. Because it can help with water retention, it's used in weight management.
- **Flax**—As we discussed in our chapter on super nutrition, this insoluble fiber is an effective bulking laxative; a source of lignins (thought to fight estrogen-related cancers); an excellent source of essential fatty acids; a digestive aid; and an appetite suppressant. Usually the seeds are ingested with a glass or two of water to relieve gas and move wastes out of the body.
- **Horsetail**—Like cleavers, horsetail is an excellent tonic for stomach ulcers, urinary tract inflammations, and damaged or inflamed tissues, again, by acting as a strong diuretic. It's a storehouse of minerals, too. Liquidize the stems or take capsules of powdered horsetail for water retention.
- **Marshmallow**—A diuretic, a laxative, a powerful anti-inflammatory, and a soothing, healing herb for the gastrointestinal tract.
- **Papaya**—The enzymes derived from the fruit and leaf aid digestion, relieve gas and bloating, and may be effective in preventing ulcers. Papaya's enzyme activity is comparable to that of pepsin and rennin, digestive enzymes useful in breaking down meat and milk proteins.
- **Peppermint**—Mint tea may be one of the most popular medicinal treatments in the world. Peppermint leaves have an oil that has been shown both to sedate the nerves and strengthen them; tone the heart muscle and

calm heart palpitations; assist in digestion; aid in nausea, seasickness, diarrhea, and spastic colon; and cure sleeplessness and nervous headache. It's often used as an overall body cleanser and tonic.

- **Plantain**—The bane of most lawn fanatics, plantain is the source of psyllium seed, used as a bulking laxative and tonic. Like flax, the seed should be consumed with plenty of water.

- **Slippery Elm**—A buffer, ideal for irritations and inflammations of the stomach, intestines, bronchials, and urinary tract. The inner bark draws out toxins and heals and soothes all mucous membranes. As an adrenal stimulant, it increases the output of blood-building substances. Slippery elm can be added to cereal or made into a gruel if swallowing a capsule is problematic.

- **Thyme**—With antiseptic, antibiotic, antispasmodic, and anaesthetic properties, thyme is an old-time remedy for stomach and bowel disorders—dyspepsia, flatulence, cramps, diarrhea, and spastic colon—as well as a tonic for throat and respiratory ailments.

- **Triphala**—As we noted earlier, this Ayurvedic formulation of three fruits is not only a gentle, effective bowel cleanser but also an overall tonic to the digestive tract and, because of its vitamin C content, an immunity booster. Often found in combination with other bowel cleansers, or with guggula (see below) for weight loss.

Circulation and Energy Boosters

- **Fenugreek**—The seeds contain substances that dissolve fatty deposits, prevent fatty accumulations, dissolve cholesterol, and relieve water retention, all of which help to free up arterial and lymphatic pathways.

- **Garlic**—Who hasn't sung the praises of this bulb? Garlic rejuvenates the body by stimulating the lymphatic system to expel waste and throw off toxins. It has been used to ward off disease and infection by boosting immunity with the antioxidants vitamin C, vitamin A, and selenium. By dissolving cholesterol and hardened plaques it opens up blood vessels and helps lower high blood pressure. It also reduces blood sugar levels. Used primarily in cooking, garlic may alternatively be chewed, or ingested in capsules or "pearls" as a dietary supplement.

• **Ginger**—An excellent circulatory stimulant. Long regarded as a digestive aid and stomach tonic, ginger is used by the Chinese to restore depleted spleen energy and get rid of excess phlegm. High in vitamins A, C, and B-complex, it's great for fending off colds and flu.

• **Gingko**—The leaves have long been used to improve circulation, but they're especially effective in promoting blood flow to the brain for improving memory and mental acuity. We find it especially helpful for both mental and physical fatigue.

• **Gotu Kola**—Otherwise known as "food for the brain," this herb appears to have an energizing, restorative effect on nerve cells, useful in instances of fatigue, nervous breakdown, and depression. It also relieves lethargy, and has been shown to enhance reflexes.

• **Guggula**—A blood purifier and circulatory stimulant, guggula is an Ayurvedic remedy. It's thought to promote flexibility and increase stamina and energy. This cousin to myrrh also stimulates the secretion of digestive juices and regular movement of the bowels.

• **Oolong tea**—Made from the partially fermented leaves of the tea bush, oolong tea may help reduce cholesterol levels and high blood pressure. Especially recommended after a rich meal.

Thyroid Activators
- **Bladderwrack**—As with all seaweeds, the iodine content of this herb stimulates metabolism, possibly because its chemical structure is similar to that of the thyroid hormone.
- **Kelp**—Rich in nearly thirty minerals, including iodine, plus vitamins A, C, E, the B-complex, and K, kelp is an important dietary supplement, as we've discussed. But it's also a metabolic stimulant and regulator, useful in burning up excess calories and keeping nutrients available for use.

Appetite Suppressants
- **Fennel**—The seeds improve digestion, take away appetite, and flush away tissue impurities by acting as a diuretic. Its Greek name, *marathron*, means "to grow thin."
- **Garcinia Cambogia**—This extract of an Indian pumpkin is widely recognized as an appetite suppressant and aid to weight loss, but it must be used consistently for at least a month before you assess its efficacy.
- **Oatstraw**—A very small amount of extract from the stems will stimulate metabolism; in larger doses, it will dampen the appetite—more so than chickweed, which is also used to treat obesity. It's indicated for indigestion, and as a tonic for the whole body.

Health Builders
- **Alfalfa**—Very rich in vitamins A, K, and D, high in trace minerals and calcium, and loaded with eight essential enzymes, this herb is typically grown as animal fodder. Its nutrients are readily absorbed and help in the assimilation of protein and calcium. Alfalfa is used as an overall tonic, helpful in eliminating excess water

and relieving urinary and bowel complaints. It's a good kidney cleanser, ulcer tonic, and fatigue reliever.

- **Astragalus**—Taken daily, this root is traditionally recognized as a powerful immune booster, used like licorice and echinacea to fend off colds. The Chinese believe it strengthens the spleen, promotes digestive energy, and strengthens chi; it does appear to raise metabolism, temper blood sugar, and increase physical energy. It's often combined with other herbs, notably ginseng and licorice, for a thoroughly rejuvenating tonic. Discontinue use at the onset of cold, flu, virus or infection.

- **Echinacea**—We'd be remiss if we didn't include this herb, one of our favorite all-round immune boosters for adults and children that should belong in every medicine cabinet. It's antiviral, antibacterial, and antifungal. Used at the beginning of any cold, flu, virus, or infection, it can help shorten the duration and lessen the intensity of the illness. There's no better blood purifier in the plant world. We do not, however, recommend that you take echinacea every day for more than a month at a time; we recommend one week on, one week off. Liquid extract in glycerine is our preference, but the herb is also available as a tincture, capsule, pill, or tea.

- **Ginseng**—Perhaps the emperor of all herbs in Chinese medicine, ginseng root stimulates and rejuvenates the cardiovascular system. It also contains substances that affect sugar metabolism, acting somewhat like insulin. Natural steroids in ginseng stimulate and regulate metabolism by acting like adrenal hormones. The root can be steamed and chewed on, or used raw and ground into a powder, or taken as a capsule or extract. Cooked in a soup with dried ginger and licorice root, it's especially warming and energizing.

- **Goldenseal**—Excellent for upper respiratory infections, particularly sore throats (gargle with it). While it has a particularly unpleasant taste, you'll thank us for it. It's recognized as an antibacterial and antiviral agent. Take it as an extract in glycerine, a tincture, or as a tea. Goldenseal is most effective when not taken every day, but only as indicated for illness. Better yet, combine with licorice and echinacea extracts.

- **Irish Moss**—Another seaweed that's a potent source of vitamins A, D, E, and K, as well as iodine, calcium, and sodium. Often used as a thyroid stimulator, it's better known for its purifying, healing, strengthening properties. Used as an appetite suppressant, too.

- **Licorice**—An extract often used to flavor candy and soothe sore throats, true licorice goes well beyond these applications: it's an adrenal stimulant, an energy booster, a mild laxative, a means of purging excess fluid and phlegm from the bronchials, an aid to circulation, a blood cleanser, a cholesterol reducer, and an anti-inflammatory. To be avoided if you have high blood pressure.

- **Nettle**—Exceptionally high in chlorophyll and iron, the leaves of this herb purify and build the blood, improve circulation, and reduce high blood pressure. Its high vitamin C content ensures that all of its iron will be absorbed; its protein and mineral content make it an excellent nutrient as well. An energizing herb—especially helpful for dieters too tired to address their weight imbalance.

- **Suma**—Extracts of the bark and root of this herb are renowned for relieving stress, restoring energy, and boosting immunity. Suma is thought to aid in metabolism.

A FINAL NOTE

Like all the other components of our program, herbs should be used in conjunction with each other to optimize their synergistic effects. They're Nature's gifts: perfectly balanced packages of healing, soothing, nourishing agents. They're ideally suited to restoring your own balance, for getting your body back into shape—your organs toned, your blood purified and strengthened, your circulation improved, your metabolism fired up, your bowels moving, your kidneys flushing. And let's reiterate: a body in balance no longer suffers the cravings that undermine health and derail efforts to lose weight. Herbs can give you the energy and the overall sense of well-being you need to transform your eating habits and remain committed to a lifetime of eating better, feeling lighter, and living to your full potential.

CHAPTER NINE

Flower Essences

Salves for the Soul

*D*riving home from her therapy session, Susan, 38, felt a panic attack come on like a Mack truck. Her chest tightened. Her heart raced. She struggled for breath. Her muscles seemed to lock up.

Instead of reaching for a Xanax—the anti-anxiety medication she'd been taking on and off for the past ten years—Susan groped in her purse and found the small vial labeled *Calming Essence* she'd picked up in the health food store. Quickly she squeezed out four drops under her tongue.

"I didn't really believe it would work," she admits. "But because I was in the car, I couldn't do what I normally do, which is to walk, take deep breaths, and wait for the Xanax to kick in. Also, the drug makes me drowsy, and I had a forty-five-minute drive ahead of me.

"Well, it worked, all right," she continues. "About twice as fast as my medication, with absolutely no side effects! In about fifteen minutes I was breathing normally and my pulse had calmed down. I couldn't believe it."

The "rescue" remedy Susan used was a combination of flower essences, substances discovered more than forty years ago to have a dramatic, tempering influence on emotionally induced ailments. Since the inception of Feeling Light, we've found flower essences extremely useful in helping our clients cope with the emotional reasons behind their weight problems. People overeat for many different reasons; we've already discussed how better nutrition and supplements can address the problem.

As our client Emily can tell you, it isn't hunger, or fatigue, or boredom, or even a love of food that makes her overeat: "It's comfort," she clarifies. "For some reason food gives me a sense of calm I desperately need and can't seem to find elsewhere."

ESSENCES AND THE MIND/BODY CONNECTION

Our approach to weight loss demands that we acknowledge the needs of the soul as well as the body. Feeling Light participant Mary Lynn suffers, as Susan does, from anxiety and depression—except that her panic attacks compel her to eat. She, too, is in therapy and on antidepressants. Yet Prozac, she found, just wasn't addressing her weight problem, despite the fact that some people claim Prozac helps stop them from overeating. So as we did with Susan, we suggested a more holistic strategy, one that took into account the emotional, as well as biochemical, reasons for destructive behavior. Our recommendations for both women: routine acupuncture treatments, meditative exercises (including, for Mary Lynn, Tai Chi and chi gong), and flower essences, including Calming Essence.

The results they report are uncannily similar. Susan's panic attacks have all but disappeared, thanks to the acupuncture, she says; for the one or two flare-ups she's had, "the Calming Essence is all I need." She keeps a vial by her bedside, "because I find that if I wake up and can't get back to sleep, a drop or two just chills me out." She's off the Xanax, which had constipated her. "All of a sudden, I feel really good," she reports. "Not sluggish. Not blah or lethargic."

And Mary Lynn, at the first sign of the panic attack that makes her reach for the nearest snack, now makes herself a cup of tea to which she adds Calming Essence. "Maybe just because it makes me sit, relax, and *stop* what I'm doing, it works," she reflects. "But I think it's helped me tap into this destressing system, so that whenever I'm upset, I can pause enough to see what's coming and stop it. It's more than appetite control. I'm not eating, because I'm not stressed out."

WHY FLOWER ESSENCES?

Emotions exert a profound influence on well-being. Studies of breast cancer victims have shown that women who attend a regular support group to air their fears and share their grief have a significantly better survival rate than those who have no such comfort source. There are those who insist, with mounting evidence to support their observation, that anxiety, fear, or depression can actually *cause* cancer—because continual stress exerts a measurable drain on the body's nutrient reservoirs, thus impairing immune response and opening the door to degenerative disease. There's literal truth in the expression, "You'll make yourself *sick with worry*": that's exactly what happens to someone suffering a panic attack, or who overeats out of emotional need.

Treating emotional causes of disease is foremost in all mind/body healing. In our experience, behavior is influenced by a constellation of influences so varied, subtle, and complex that controlling or modifying it can be equally varied, subtle, and complex. Emotional well-being is a delicate balance, one not achieved simply by the introduction of synthetic chemicals and hormones. The human psyche cannot be mapped out, probed, rewired, sewn together, and cured with pills.

Which is why we overwhelmingly favor flower essences. They're gentle, noninvasive, and utterly natural. And from what our clients tell us, they're utterly effective.

WHAT ARE THEY?

Flower essences were the lifetime achievement of Dr. Edward Bach, a medical doctor and homeopath who practiced in London during the first quarter of this century. The more patients he treated, the more convinced he became that "the primary diseases of man are such defects as pride, cruelty, hate, self-centeredness, ignorance, instability and greed." Over and over he noted that a patient's personality, attitude, and outlook had more to do with recovery than any procedure or drug he could administer. In 1930, Bach left London for the Welsh countryside, where he pursued and perfected the remedies for which he would become famous. Derived from thirty-eight flowers—the petals or blooms only—Bach's flower essences addressed a similarly broad spectrum of human emotions, from passivity to aggression, despair to pride, uncertainty to resignation. Since his death in 1936, more essences have been discovered to address still other personality traits.

—How Do They Work?—

The very dilute "essence" of an herb or flower can have a catalytic effect on the human body, prompting natural healing mechanisms to take over. Flower essences work by tempering the patient's emotional extremes, neither obliterating nor exaggerating the predominant symptom. For example, a person characterized by intensity or hyperactivity might find those same qualities translated into steady, purposeful energy by taking the essence derived from the bloom of the vervain plant. To use an image we introduced early on, flower essences create the dynamic equilibrium illustrated by the yin yang symbol.

The Catalytic Effect of Essences

An occupational therapist will tell you that helping the elderly, the impaired, or the severely injured to function normally is an inexact science requiring a variety of approaches. The catalyst may be to get them involved in arts and crafts, such as woodworking, painting, or sculpture. Therapy may be physical or recreational—playing volleyball or going bowling. It may be quietly reflective: listening to music, wandering through a museum, taking a walk in the woods.

The occupational therapist recognizes that patients have it within themselves to be healed. It's merely a matter of hitting upon the right stimulus to turn feelings of pain, fear, or despair into energy, confidence, and ambition.

Flower essences work in much the same way. They're catalysts. Bach believed that each flower's vital energies could stir up or free energies blocked by negative emotion. Much as acupuncture uses needles to stimulate and un-block chi, the essential life force nourishing our every cell, Bach used flower essences to awaken the positive corollar-ies to negative emotional traits. Day by day, with regular dosing, a subtle but noticeable transformation takes place.

WHICH ONES SHOULD I TAKE?

While we'd encourage you to try any of the thirty-eight as indicated for emotional need, we've selected five (in ad-dition to Calming Essence) that have proven especially ef-fective, when taken together as a formula, in treating the imbalances that lead to emotional eating. You'll probably recognize aspects of yourself in at least one—but most likely all—of the following descriptions:

Agrimony

THE ESSENCE: derived from the field flower whose blooms are short-lived, small, and yellow. They grow in tall, con-ical spikes.

PERSONALITY PROFILE: You're Doris Day. You're the per-ennial optimist. You're the life of the party, the person everyone wants around because you're always cheerful and so . . . *together*. In fact, whenever anyone asks how you are, you say "Fine!" enthusiastically—because you'd like to believe it. Your friends think nothing ever gets to you. You enjoy having them think that. The truth is. . . .

The truth is something so painful, so awful, so shameful, you can't face it, and so you continue to put on a happy face and drown your torment secretly, furtively, in food. Half the time you don't even know why you eat, except that it feels good. Nurturing. Comforting. Food is like a salve or blanket, smothering out the needy voice of your malnourished soul. It's your best friend, literally, since none of the people you call friends really know you, really know what's eating you, really ever see the real you. *You* don't even see or know the real you. You've been holding it all inside for so long that the burden and toxicity of it makes you literally ache—and you thought it was arthritis.

Agrimony has been called the truth serum, for it helps bring out into the open whatever you've been hiding, even from yourself. Financial or relationship troubles, feelings of shame, or stifled emotion can be addressed and resolved. For the first time, you can step back from your life of constant distraction without fear of the person you'll find at its center. You can let go of your burdens. You can admit them to others. You can enjoy true intimacy without fear of the other person discovering something loathsome or hateful. You accept yourself. With the demons exorcised, you have no need to feed them. That ready smile you've been flashing at everybody for years is no longer a mask: It's *you*.

Cherry Plum
THE ESSENCE: derived from the pure white, five-petaled flower of a shrub that's often planted in rows as a windbreak.

PERSONALITY PROFILE: I eat too much, I know, and I've got to stop, but I just . . . can't! I start eating and I can't stop! I'm out of control!

It's terrifying, but there it is. You're out of control in your habits, whether it's food, or alcohol, or cigarettes, or pills, or exercise, or even crash diets.

Anorexic or obese, you've got a control thing: control is really, really important, and yet, instead of being in control, you're in the grip of something overwhelming, something beyond your power to stop or moderate. You binge. You starve. You diet, but never for very long. It seems like the more you need self-discipline, the more likely you are to lose it entirely.

Cherry Plum is for you, whether you're way out of control or just frequently and easily overwhelmed by the tasks before you—including losing the pounds those binges keep plastering on. You're probably suffering from hypertension or elevated cholesterol. Frequently, you can't sleep. You're a mess, you admit—but instead of correcting the problem, you go on a bender that makes it even worse.

Cherry Plum is the place to begin. It eases that tension gripping you like a vise and driving you to compulsive, destructive acts. It gives you the composure you need to exert self-discipline. You'll feel courage instead of despair, peace of mind where before, stress drove you to excess. You can see an attack of self-sabotage coming—and you'll have the self-confidence to disarm it. Cherry Plum gives you the strength and discipline you need to fast, to cleanse, to start over . . . and to stick with the program.

Crab Apple
THE ESSENCE: derived from the white, pink, or red flowers of the tree characterized by its gnarled branches and small, applelike fruits.

PERSONALITY PROFILE: Are you a neatnik? Are you compulsive about your hygiene, your hair, your house? Are you sick and tired of being five or ten pounds overweight? Are you ever completely satisfied with *anything*?

Admit it: you're not. You really feel your floor could be cleaner, your kids could be more polite, your cupboards could be more organized. You honestly feel like the only thing between you and true happiness are those troublesome pounds that make waistbands roll, or those hip pads that make pants fit funny, or that cellulite that dimples the backs of your thighs, or . . . need we go on? There's always something. You're not perfect, and it bugs you. The world is not perfect, and it drives you nuts. Your day can be ruined by hair that won't curl right or a picture that won't hang straight. You can't even breathe without noticing all the particles in the air, particles that make your allergies flare.

Fortunately, there's Crab Apple. It's a source of peace you'll never find elsewhere. It grants you personal satisfaction in the likelihood you'll never grant it to yourself. It shows you the beauty the world has to offer, despite your insistence on seeing all the imperfections. It frees you from obsessing over details by showing you the big picture—where you're happy and loved for who you are, imperfect though you may be.

Crab Apple will feel like a tonic, because it is. In conjunction with fasting or a cleansing program, this essence is an excellent detoxifier. You'll find it offers the sense of purity you crave.

Gentian

THE ESSENCE: derived from the showy bluish-purple or even crimson flowers of the biennial, which grows in dry hilly pastures or in dunes or cliffs.

PERSONALITY PROFILE: You're trying. Really, you are. You're trying to lose weight, but it's just not working. It's not working because nothing ever does. You're not going to attempt to fast, though; you just know you'll fail. And you certainly don't believe in weird holistic cures like *flower essences*.

Skeptical, pessimistic, easily discouraged, and at root convinced of failure, you're exactly the person to benefit from this essence—and probably a number of others. You greet every challenge with negative resignation, with a big sigh that says, Well, I'll give it a try, *but* . . .

Permanent weight loss is a challenge that is full of ups and downs, with periods of success punctuated by small setbacks. When those setbacks are discouraging enough to prompt you to quit trying altogether, Gentian is the essence that can help restore your confidence and encourage you to believe enough in success to try again. In concert with other supportive measures—getting positive group encouragement, for example—Gentian can provide the can-do attitude, the fortitude, and the perseverance you need to resolve difficulties, embrace challenges, and succeed on the heels of failure. It's the essence of resilience, which for you may just prove to be the key to getting off weight "plateaus" and sticking to long-term goals to achieve permanent balance.

Walnut
THE ESSENCE: derived from both the male and female blooms that precede the leaves on this tall, nut-bearing tree.

PERSONALITY PROFILE: Change is the undercurrent of all life: no growth of any kind is possible without it. And yet, you can't bear to turn over a new leaf; you can barely stand to have your furniture rearranged. You like what's familiar, what feels like a well-worn glove, what is as reflexive as breathing. That's the privilege of age, right? All those hard learning phases are past. Or so you'd like to think.

Walnut is the essence that enables transition, whether you're struggling to adapt to a new job, a new home, a new relationship, a birth, a death—or a new set of dietary habits. It's not that you necessarily *like* your current habits, but you can't quite bring yourself to break with them. Maybe you're simply lacking the courage to heed your own drummer and you succumb too readily to what other people envision for you. You need a little boost, a little reassurance, a little confidence. You need Walnut essence.

Walnut is especially useful for tuning into that voice that says, "It's time for a *real* change." It can also help you tune out all those well-meaning but negative friends, family, or colleagues who keep offering advice. You'll have a clear picture of what you want, where you're going, and how to get there. Walnut can help you find the courage you didn't think you had to make lasting, healthful changes in the way you eat and in the way you relate to food.

Calming Essence
A combination of five essences, including:

- **Star of Bethlehem** for emotional shock and physical trauma;
- **Rock Rose** for terror, and the panic arising from fear;
- **Impatiens** for irritability and anger;
- **Cherry Plum** for loss of control;
- **Clematis** for lack of mental focus.

As we've indicated, Calming Essence is appropriate for dealing with acute stress, fear, pain, shock, sorrow, panic attacks, temper tantrums—or any emotional, physical, or mental crisis that drives you to seek relief in food, alcohol, cigarettes, or drugs. The combination of essences relieves pain, tempers the emotional excess that makes you lose control, and restores calm, clear thinking. It may be taken daily, or as indicated by a crisis.

HOW DO I TAKE THEM?

Bach found that merely holding a petal of impatiens helped to calm and soothe him. For his less intuitive patients, however, he developed tinctures that preserved the vital essences he had experienced in the field. The flower is steeped in water to extract its essence, and then the essence is suspended in alcohol (brandy from grapes, to be exact). It's typically administered by mouth: Place four drops under your tongue, taking care not to touch the dropper to any part of your mouth, as contamination with saliva may destroy the essence left in the bottle.

Likewise, the drops may be taken as a "tea," in hot water. Putting the essence in hot water evaporates the alcohol after twenty minutes, which may be preferable for those who want to avoid alcohol altogether. We also urge our clients to try rubbing a few drops directly into their skin—on the inside of the wrists, on the temples, behind the ears, or under the arms. Many find the essences most effective when added to bathwater: Put twenty drops in a tubful of hot water and soak for twenty minutes.

Consistency and regularity are the keys to effectiveness. We urge our clients to put a dropperful in an eight-ounce glass of water and sip from the glass throughout the day. The essences are especially useful in weight management when used in conjunction with other healing practices, such as acupressure or acupuncture, meditation, Tai Chi and chi gong, or yoga.

What will you feel? Possibly an immediate sense of relief, or as Cheryl, 36, describes it, "an absence of that edge that makes you focus on food." Cheryl adds a dropperful from each of the five essences we've described to a large water bottle, every day, as part of her strategy to stay off medication, caffeine, and unhealthy snacks. "The day I accidentally left them in my car, they were sorely missed," she says. "I felt a drastic difference in how the stress of my work affected me."

On the other hand, you may feel nothing—at first. Our client Madelyne had been combining essences without noticing much of anything until she decided she could benefit most from Crab Apple. ("I'm the kind of person who picks up a broom to do some sweeping when I'm at a *friend's* house," she confides.) She put two dropperfuls of Crab Apple in a glass of water, which she sipped throughout the day, and eliminated the other essences.

"The whole day seemed more relaxed," she insists. "I didn't go on one of my snack hunts. Usually around three or four in the afternoon, when the kids come home from school and want a snack, I have one too, 'cause my energy's low and I can't take a nap. But the essence took away that needy feeling. I felt fine—calmer, somehow."

Madelyne's experience is probably typical: she was skeptical, she was resistant, but once she tried them, she was a total convert. We know people who've been shopping at health food stores for years who say, "Oh, sure, I've seen those bottles—but I've never tried them." We know of nothing quite as simple or effective as these little secrets, these flower essence gems. They're safe. They're gentle. They can't hurt you, even if you take ones that are inappropriate for you.

If you recognize yourself in a few of them, try mixing up your own formulation. They're not a medication; you can use them indefinitely, with absolutely no side effects.

They're *transformational*, which means they certainly deserve a place in our program, and in your life. They're Nature's way of helping us attain balance in our emotional lives—a critical strategy when it comes to managing weight and overcoming self-destructive, unhealthy habits.

CHAPTER TEN

Triggering Homeostasis

How Acupuncture and Acupressure Facilitate Weight Management

*N*ancy, 45, loves exercise. A physical education teacher by profession, she's also dedicated to the gym in her leisure, doing step aerobics, stationary biking, and vigorous walking four times a week. Yet surprisingly, she's overweight—over 200 pounds. She's carrying the weight she gained for her third child, and then some. Exercise doesn't budge it.

"I was a chubby baby," Nancy insists, "and a compulsive eater. Food was my security, my way of rewarding myself for always being the good girl." Weight was *always an issue in her house. One of her earliest memories was watching her mother eat out of a half-gallon container of ice cream, standing at the kitchen counter watching "I Love Lucy"—but then insisting that bread was a no-no for herself and her daughters. "I craved bread," says Nancy. "I craved sweets. I craved all the greasy, salty foods—especially french fries."*

But since she started Feeling Light, that's all changed. The weight is starting to budge. She can see it in the mirror; she can feel it in her clothes; she can see it in her skin. It's been easy, losing the twenty pounds she estimates she's dropped in two months, because, she says, "I'm not being controlled by food any more. I'm not gravitating toward it, I'm not even thinking about it. I don't have the cravings I used to. I just got back from a wedding where I told myself I could have anything I wanted, and you know what? I had veggies without the dip. I had capon stuffed with rice and didn't eat the capon. It wasn't like I said, 'Oh, you shouldn't have that.' I didn't want it. Now for me, that's simply incredible."

What was responsible for this transformation?

"The acupuncture and acupressure," says Nancy. "I get those points in my ear stimulated, and I notice an immediate reaction in my hunger pangs. What they say is true: feel good, and you'll lose the weight. Well, I feel really good after stimulating those ear points, and that's why these pounds are finally coming off."

ANCIENT ART, MODERN SCIENCE

Acupuncture, or the insertion of fine needles at different places on the skin, is a practice as ancient as recorded history. It was the outgrowth, and refinement, of a healing touch we now term *acupressure*—using one's fingers to exert pressure on places observed to stimulate or calm various nerves, muscles, organs, and systems of the human body. Other Eastern modalities, such as shiatsu, address imbalances in the body similarly, by stimulating these points.

The points themselves are gateways to the life energy or bioelectricial current the Chinese call *chi*, the Japanese call *ki*, the Koreans call *qi*, the Indians call *prana*, the Tibetans call *rlun*, and Wilhelm Reich termed *"orgone energy."* Chi runs along circuits or pathways called meridians, fourteen of which can be mapped on the human body, extending from the crown of the head to the tips of the toes and fingers. The Chinese believe that pain, numbness, behavioral disorders, mental illness, and disease are all manifestations of a disruption in the flow of chi along these meridians. Through acupuncture or acupressure, an excess of chi can be dispersed, and a deficiency can be corrected by eliminating blockages that occur along the meridians. For more than 4,000 years, healers have treated maladies of body and mind by pinpointing these blockages and stimulating them to free up the flow of chi. There are 365 so-called main acupoints whereby a skilled practitioner can access chi and restore balance to the body.

It is no mere coincidence that these acupoints happen also to correspond to the motor points of muscles, nerve trigger points, and the nerve trunks themselves. The effect of stimulating these points—whether with fingers, needles, or electrodes—has been measured by Western scientists in red and white blood cell count, immunoglobulin levels, EEG and EKG tracings, bronchodilation, hemoglobin levels, digestive enzyme production, and endorphin activity. It is thought that acupuncture and acupressure work by stimulating the sympathetic and parasympathetic nervous systems, effectively triggering the body's own powerful healing mechanisms. Certainly by spurring the release of endorphins—narcotic-like chemicals the body manufactures in response to pain or stress—both acupuncture and acupressure have proven to be effective in pain and stress management, appetite suppression, and addiction with-

---

—ACUPUNCTURE—

Many people are timid about receiving acupuncture due to fear of needles. In actuality, the experience is pleasurable, relaxing, and surprisingly painless. Acupuncture needles are extremely fine, made of stainless steel, and solid, unlike other needles which are hollow. They neither draw anything away nor eject anything into the body. Because they are thin and inserted quickly, you barely feel them.

In Feeling Light we encourage our clients to try acupuncture at the hands of a licensed health professional or licensed practitioner. (Of course, do not try performing acupuncture on your own.) Clients who have followed our advice experience how the stimulation of select sites can ease pain, induce deep relaxation, and offer relief from the nagging, ceaseless voice of craving. Many of our Feeling Light participants are drawn to the program precisely because they've experienced the dramatic impact that acupuncture can have on weight loss and on everything from carpal tunnel syndrome to degenerative bone disease, from asthma to urinary tract infection, from fatigue to hypothyroidism.

Refer to our appendix for help in finding a board certified acupuncturist near you.

drawal. Addictions to nicotine, cocaine, and alcohol have been successfully treated with acupuncture at more than twenty hospital-supervised substance abuse centers nationwide, with efficacy rates as high as 85 percent.

Little wonder, then, that so many who are suffering from eating disorders or obesity have turned to these ancient Oriental practices for help in curbing their compulsive habits regarding food. Acupressure in particular is simple, economic, devoid of side effects—and documented to be effective in 70 to 80 percent of obesity cases studied worldwide.

ACUPRESSURE AND AURICULOTHERAPY

We are well aware that not everyone has access to an acupuncturist, so we also stress that with a little practice, our participants can enjoy similar relief at their own hands. We teach them acupressure because not everyone is comfortable with the idea of needles and not everyone wants to run to a practitioner the moment a craving strikes or a binge threatens. Acupressure is easy, accessible, free of cost, immediate in effect, and effective in weight control. Its success lies in its ability to strengthen willpower while nipping cravings in the bud.

Specifically, we teach our clients to apply pressure to the acupoints in their ears.

Why the ears? For centuries, cultures from the East and Middle East have stapled, pierced, burned, and bloodlet places on the ear for addressing problems as varied as infertility and conjunctivitis. The Chinese have always recognized the importance of the ear in terms of its acupoints, because the ear is the external correlate to the kidneys, which are the seat of ancestral chi, and because all fourteen meridians have representation there. In 1957, a Frenchman by the name of Paul Nogier noted that the acupoints on the ear correlated almost exactly to the body's major organs and nerve centers if one were to envision the ear as a human fetus *in utero*—upside down, as in the womb.

This startling observation led mainland China to explore anew the efficacy of treating imbalance by stimulating ear points alone. Researchers found that by stimulating ear points of the vagus or parasympathetic nerve, the nerve that helps regulate functions such as heartbeat and digestion, they could treat patients with hypertension, hyperglycemia, coronary heart disease, edema, and other life-threatening complications of obesity. Their ongoing success has prompted us to adopt this particular adaptation of acupuncture, called auriculotherapy, as one of many tools we employ in Feeling Light. In our experience, clients who combine it with proper diet, exercise, meditative and breathing exercises, and nutritional herbs and supplements reap the greatest benefits.

THE PRESSURE POINTS

In addition to the sympathetic nerve point, we've zeroed in on seven other spots that facilitate weight loss by curbing cravings, lessening appetite, relieving stress, strengthening willpower, and improving metabolic function. Acupressure on these ear points effectively diminishes overactive bodily functions (adrenaline release, for example), while at the same time it increases sluggish physiological functions (insulin or thyroxin production, for instance). A study conducted at the Nanjing College of Traditional Chinese Medicine in Nanjing, China, found that in fifty cases of obesity, stimulation of mouth, spleen, stomach, and sympathetic points on the ear curbed compulsive eating in all but three of the patients. Another re-

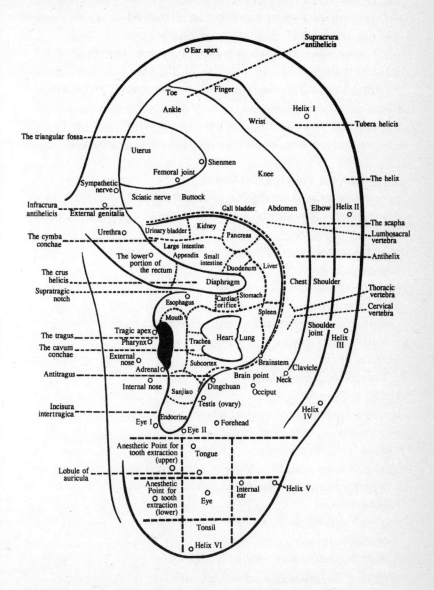

EAR CHART SHOWING POINTS FOR THE ENTIRE BODY.

searcher found that in twenty-four overweight patients, stimulation of the stomach point alone led to an average weight loss of 14.5 pounds over eight weeks.

You can perform acupressure on yourself or on another. First, acquaint yourself with the landscape of the ear. Use a mirror to examine your own ear, or work with a spouse or friend. Study the diagram we've included here in simplified form: see if you can find each point on your own ear or on someone else's ear. From top to bottom the points are:

Shenmen (or Neurogate) Point
  • acts as potent analgesic or anaesthetic
  • induces relaxation
  • eases anxiety
  • lifts depression
Stomach Point
  • alleviates stress
  • relieves insomnia
  • relieves indigestion, peptic ulcers, and gas
  • addresses eating disorders
Mouth Point
  • targets eating disorders
Hunger Point
  • diminishes hunger and appetite
  • increases sensation of fullness
  • addresses compulsive eating
  • facilitates weight loss
  • helps regulate blood sugar levels
Kidney Point
  • strengthens willpower
  • boosts metabolism
  • strengthens and tonifies kidneys
  • relieves lethargy
  • relieves headache
  • builds blood

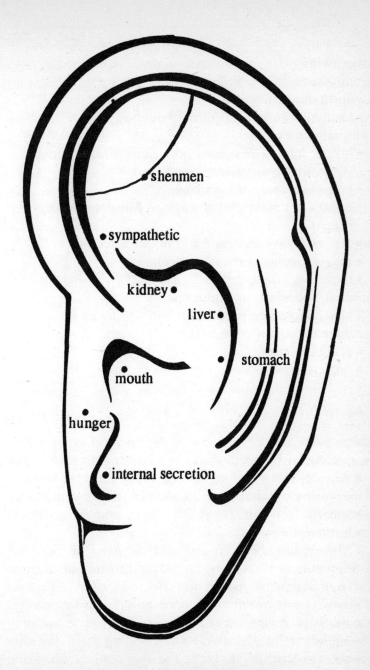

EAR POINTS FOR WEIGHT MANAGEMENT.

Liver Point
- improves liver's ability to filter out toxins, and store and release nutrients
- facilitates flow of chi throughout body

Sympathetic Point
- brings into homeostasis both sympathetic and para-sympathetic nervous systems
- improves vascular circulation
- improves uptake and absorption functions of digestive organs
- acts as strong analgesic and organ relaxant
- relieves stomach spasm and ulcers
- improves bile secretion

Internal Secretion (or Endocrine)
- affects hormone production and endocrine system
- improves digestive function
- boosts metabolism
- improves excretion

HOW TO DO IT

Acupressure can be done every day, several times a day, or as dictated by need. Begin by choosing an ear—either ear will do, but only one should be probed per session. Wipe your ear carefully with alcohol. Wash your hands thoroughly; you can use your nails or your fingertips to apply pressure.

Always use shenmen and add as many of the other seven points as you desire. Our typical treatments include a total of five points. Each point selected should be pressed and held one or two minutes, once daily, for lasting clinical benefit. Bear in mind that the points themselves are only one millimeter in diameter, so that finding them day after day is a matter of studying the diagram, familiarizing yourself with the ear you'll be working on, and paying very close attention to feelings of tenderness or increased sensitivity. An active reflex point—one that is increasingly sensitive to applied pressure—is not only your clue that you've found the right spot but also that the point's corresponding organ or nervous system is truly in need of healing. Tenderness and sensitivity should abate as healing progresses. Alternate the ear you stimulate daily.

What to Expect

Here's what our Feeling Light participants who've tried acupressure on their ears report:

- deep relaxation
- sensation of satisfied hunger
- sensation of lightness
- deeper, more restful sleep
- better coping skills
- fewer cravings
- less compulsive eating
- fewer headaches
- better elimination
- improved outlook and attitude

"It knocked off my craving for sugar like nothing I've ever seen," says Emily, the teacher who works with the learning disabled. *"When I was confronted on Halloween with ten free pounds of chocolate, I had raspberries instead!"*

Occupational therapist Debbie says she isn't tired anymore. "I don't know whether it's the acupressure or the vitamins I'm taking," she observes, "but I feel like I have a lot more energy. I think I used to eat just out of fatigue, because I looked to food to perk me up, give me energy."

Jackie, 38, a family therapist, did twenty minutes of acupuncture in her left ear and lost her appetite for two days running. "It's made me relearn how to eat," she says. "I do my Smoothie, I do my acupressure, and I eat less!"

"Just because you can't explain something doesn't mean it doesn't work," says Mike, 32, a software engineer. "You don't have to believe in all this chi stuff to have it work for you. I don't question it anymore. I just do it, and I feel a whole lot better."

CHAPTER ELEVEN

Tai Chi Chuan

Tapping the Spring of Eternal Youth

This is something they do in California, right?

Tie chee what?

Oh, no, not me. Not martial arts. No meditation mumbo-jumbo, either.

I already do aerobics. Or I'm going to, just as soon as I lose some of this weight.

Be honest: you had planned to skip this chapter, right?

*   *   *

Well, don't. Because chances are, you have no idea what you're missing. Tai Chi Chuan, or Tai Chi for short, may sound weird, mystical, foreign, New Agey, or otherwise something you don't see yourself doing in your living room, but if ever there was an easy, painless cure for what ails you, *this is it.*

You don't need to be a Zen master, a practicing Buddhist, or a Taoist monk. Nor do you need to buy clingy little Lycra outfits, a health club membership, a stair exerciser, or Rollerblades. Tai Chi is something you can do right now, wherever you are, whatever your age or condition. You can be old, overweight, completely out of shape, inflexible, arthritic, or utterly skeptical, and Tai Chi will work for you, increasing energy and agility, replacing fat with muscle tone, and tempering emotional imbalance. Or you can be young and athletic—and still find it challenging to the body and tonifying to the soul.

You can reap these benefits immediately, however slowly or uncertainly you perform the movements we're going to detail here. If you're already doing some of the exercises we detailed earlier (see Chapter 3, Readying the Body), don't stop: just start incorporating a few Tai Chi repetitions. The more you practice, the more its circular movements, rhythmic breathing exercises, and flowing postures will become second nature, something as vital to your well-being as eating and sleeping. The more innate Tai Chi becomes, the more you are likely to see and feel its long-term mental and physical effects: younger-looking skin, all-over flexibility, balance, coordination, agility, stamina, strength, better concentration, sharper mental focus, self-confidence, and emotional composure. Imagine if you could combine a chiropractic adjustment, a shiatsu massage, a yoga session, and meditation into one mind/body "exercise": that exercise is Tai Chi.

Tai Chi is a system of movement and breathing designed to prevent illness and promote longevity—ostensibly the goals of Western exercise. Except there is nothing pounding, strenuous, straining, exhausting, or winding about Tai Chi Chuan. The same cannot be said for aerobics, jogging, weight lifting, mountain biking, or any of a number of fitness activities or sports that seize popular fancy. That's the whole problem with exercise in America: it's least practicable for those who need it most. The old, the infirm, and the overweight are easily deterred, if not outright repelled, by activities seemingly designed for the youthful, the athletic, and the healthy. No wonder so many Americans are literally dying from inactivity.

Which is why we're particularly keen about getting you to put aside your reticence and give this a try.

Tai Chi Chuan, technically speaking, is a Chinese martial art. It was the brainchild of a thirteenth-century Taoist monk who, witnessing a fight between a snake and a crane, was impressed by how the snake defeated its much more powerful opponent through circular, evasive movements, ultimately ensnaring the bird in its coils. Tai Chi is the softer, "internal" version of kung fu. Both develop combative readiness, but whereas kung fu develops the bones, muscles, and outer physique, Tai Chi concerns itself with cultivating, accumulating, and directing chi, the vital energy that flows through all living things. To have control over one's chi is to harness a formidable power: the body is poised, both mentally and physically, to anticipate and deflect any aggression by gathering and projecting concentrated, internal energy.

Tai Chi is frequently practiced in concert with chi gong, a system of breathing exercises also devoted to the development of chi. It's almost impossible to perform the movements of one without incorporating tenets of the other. The circular, repetitive motions of Tai Chi are executed in tempo with slow inhalations and exhalations; in chi gong exercises, the breathing is the primary focus. Often participants in our class will say, "But I'm concentrating so hard on remembering the moves I can't remember to breathe right!" We tell them not to worry; getting the moves down is indeed the first priority in learning Tai Chi, and more often than not, the breathing falls into place as the moves become rote. But that's why we also incorporate some chi gong exercises, because they help our students acquire the breathing habits that will ultimately make Tai Chi the moving meditation, the harmonization of body and mind, sinew and breath, that it was intended to be. Gentle, deep breathing combined with controlled yet flowing movements gives the practitioner a sense of peace and strength, relaxation and readiness. We can think of no Western equivalent, no exercise as holistic in nature or as healing in effect.

WHAT IT CAN DO FOR YOU

"You think, 'It's so slow, it can't be doing anything'— but it is!" insists Susan, 38, a massage therapist who signed up for our class after finding acupuncture helpful for an old hip injury.

What Susan has noticed—and what her clients have remarked upon—is that ever since she started doing Tai Chi, her massage technique has improved. And she's much less fatigued by her work.

"If I stand at my massage table and bend from my waist, with my knees straight, I feel it in my back," she explains, "whereas if I bend my knees a little, with my feet apart, and step into a move, like we do in class, then there's more of a flow. Energy's coming from below my waist, where I've consciously centered it. My clients feel the difference. They think I've changed my technique. 'You're more refined, somehow,' one woman told me."

*   *   *

Lou, 52, a high school teacher, already knew what it meant to channel chi: he'd taken yoga years ago. He was also familiar with the physicality of the martial arts, having been a karate enthusiast in his early thirties. But the "ego thing, the accomplishment aspect of karate" no longer appealed to him; at this point in his life, Lou says, "I wanted the spiritual aspect—that meditational release from the world and all its pressures." Without fail, now, Lou attends our weekly class. "There are those evenings where I feel down, where I don't feel up to getting out and doing something—and that's when I make sure I get there," he explains, "because I know when I get out of class, I'll feel elated.

"It's the release that comes from being totally lost in something," he adds. "If I played the piano, it'd be the same thing. In no way is it a burden, a chore, a task. I'm happy participating in it."

The physical and mental benefits of Tai Chi have in some instances been quantified. A study sponsored by the American Medical Association found that Tai Chi measurably improved balance and coordination among the elderly, reducing the incidence of falls among 2,328 senior citizens by 25 percent. A study conducted at the Research Institute for Sports Medicine in Beijing found that people who practiced Tai Chi had better skeleto-muscular fitness and a higher rate of metabolism than those who didn't exercise. Tai Chi has also been shown to lower blood pressure in hypertensive patients because its motions replicate the cardiovascular workout of swimming or dancing.

Its most profound effects on well-being, however, cannot be measured—only articulated by those who've experienced them.

"Never in my life have I been what you'd call athletic or coordinated," says Susan. "I was never into fitness. But I've found

that with Tai Chi, if you can get beyond the initial 'I feel really stupid,' or, 'This is so slow, it can't be working' phase—then you get to feel really balanced. It brings all the edges of scatteredness together. You're like one ball of energy."

"There've been times when I got high playing basketball," reflects Lou. "Something about the flow of the game, the running, the back and forth, the up and down, the team work, a perfect pass. That's what chi feel like. There's a healthy rightness to it, a sensation of motion where everything is falling into place. Now I can tap into that just walking down the street. I'm basically healthy because my mental outlook is healthy, because my chi is flowing."

GETTING STARTED

We're going to give you a taste of what Tai Chi and chi gong feel like by giving you four different things to practice: a meditation, two chi gong exercises, and a Tai Chi exercise for long life. There are in fact many different Tai Chi forms, the legacy of several different families, and there are literally hundreds of chi gong exercises. But even a Tai Chi master will perform with regularity only a few out of the vast repertoire. The value of any given form lies in its repetition, in performing the series of movements over and over, in practicing one method of breathing until it is second nature.

Learning Tai Chi is in many ways like learning dance moves; it helps to have a choreographer by your side, giving you feedback. But there's no reason you can't pick up some of the basic moves here: the four exercises we've chosen to detail are those we feel anyone can benefit by doing, however imperfectly. We'll feel we have succeeded if, in adopting these moves, you're intrigued enough to sign up for a class or get a hold of our video (see Appendix).

- Start out by giving yourself a chunk of free time—ten to twenty minutes. Unplug the phone or turn off the ringer and have your machine set to answer. Don't be anticipating any errands that you have to do. Pick a time when you're not likely to receive visitors, either— we find first thing in the morning best. Make sure there are no radios, televisions, computers, or other sources of background noise audible—unless it's the sound of birds singing or wind in the trees. Weather permitting, we encourage you to practice out-of-doors; indeed, if you went to Beijing (or even Golden Gate park in San Francisco), you'd see young and old performing Tai Chi in trancelike quiet in the parks.
- Don't chew gum. Wear flat-soled, comfortable shoes such as sneakers. Wear loose clothing. Take a few minutes to calm down, to even out your breathing, to void your thoughts.
- Voiding your thoughts can, of course, be easier said than done, especially if you're not in the habit of meditating. It seems the harder you try not to think about something, the more insistently it occupies your mind. This is to be expected, at least at first. Fear not: while Tai Chi is best executed in a state of calm, it's also the perfect thing to bestow calm when you can't banish distracting thoughts or emotions. The movements themselves require such concentration to perform that you won't be able to think of anything but the exact positioning and coordination of your limbs. You'll be newly conscious of how your body occupies space. You'll also become extremely conscious of your inhalations and exhalations. In short, if you have trouble clearing your mind prior to Tai Chi, be assured you'll get the knack in the practice itself.

TAN TIEN MEDITATION

Our suggestion is to start your session with a meditative exercise designed to help you not only rein in your thoughts but also to tune into your chi. It's a good way to end a Tai Chi session, too. In fact, it's a good meditation to perform anywhere, anytime, whether you're sitting down, lying down, or standing and need a little respite from the pressures or thoughts tying you in knots.

Rest your hands on your lower abdomen so that your fingertips are positioned about two inches below your navel (Figure 1). This spot is what the Chinese call your lower *tan tien*, one of three collecting points for circulating chi. It's thought that this tan tien in particular is the locus of healing; if you can center your thoughts and energy here, then you can restore tranquility, promote healing, and bolster your health.

As you rest your fingertips on this point, rest your mind's eye there also. Imagine your abdomen as a balloon, a balloon you want to fill with chi. Breathe in through your nose, allowing your abdomen—not your chest—to expand. Imagine this expansion to be chi rushing in to your tan tien. As you exhale, imagine you are releasing chi out of the balloon to energize your whole body. Or concentrate on speeding it directly to those places where you're in need of healing. Repeat this deep, healing breath two more times before allowing your normal breathing pattern to resume. Continue to concentrate on your tan tien. You may unconsciously find yourself taking another deep, abdominal breath. The cycle of three deep inhalations and exhalations can be repeated every three to five minutes if you find you want to continue with this meditation.

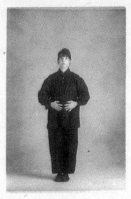

FIGURE 1

ABOUT BREATHING

One thing is for sure: Tai Chi will improve your breathing, so that you get more oxygen out of every inhalation and void more carbon dioxide in every exhalation. Slower, deeper, longer respiration will improve your lung capacity, sharpen your mental powers, massage and nourish internal organs, promote digesion and nutrient absorption, and cultivate chi. You'll have more energy, while at the same time you'll feel more relaxed.

There are basically two breathing techniques, one the reverse of the other. The most intuitive is called natural abdominal breathing, where you allow your abdomen to expand when you inhale, and deflate when you exhale. Reversed abdominal breathing is exactly that. Whatever technique you adopt, bear in mind that it will take practice before you can do it without thinking about it. Always breathe in and out through your nose.

UNIVERSAL LIFE POST

A form of standing meditation, Universal Life Post is a chi gong exercise that incorporates both the relaxed posture and the deep breathing we've just discussed. The breathing helps you achieve a meditative state whereby you can accumulate chi in your lower tan tien; the standing posture allows chi to flow at your direction, washing away physical tension. The longer you stand, the deeper you'll go into a state of relaxation and transcendence from everyday stress. Concentrate on utterly relaxing your frame, as if it were suspended from above; focus your attention on your breathing, taking pains to slow it down, to allow it to expand your lungs and move your abdomen. Give yourself plenty of time. The result? Your mind will be freed of extraneous thoughts; your body will be freed of impediments blocking the flow of chi.

Start by assuming the relaxed stance we've detailed. With 90 percent of your weight on one foot, extend your other leg forward and rest it lightly, heel raised off the ground.

Now extend your arms at shoulder height and hold them out there as if you were holding a large ball at arms' length. One hand—the hand over your extended foot—will exceed the reach of the other by about two inches (Figure 2).

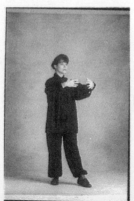

FIGURE 2 (LEFT VIEW)

Stand in this position, breathing deeply and gently, as long as you can, anywhere from five to thirty minutes (Figure 3).

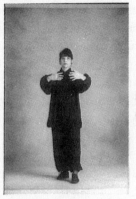

FIGURE 3
(FRONTAL VIEW)

Now switch the placement of your feet and assume the same meditative stance for equally long. While standing, concentrate on an imaginary circle that runs from the top of your head to your feet, around your arms and shoulders. Think about trying to fill this circle as you breathe, expanding yourself with each breath. Focus on the oneness of your body, united by this circle. Such imagery may help you relax and remain balanced (Figure 4).

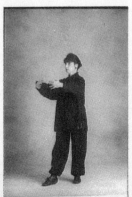

FIGURE 4
(RIGHT VIEW)

Or, focus your mind on your tan tien. The Yellow Emperor's Canon of Internal Medicine, China's most ancient and revered healing text, says that "Genuine chi attends on a tranquil mind that is clear of extravagant desires, and disease will never come around when chi is concentrated in the tan tien region."

Think of your chi accumulating just below your navel. Imagine, perhaps, that your entire body is a balloon, filling up with chi with each inhalation, expanding with chi equally in all directions as you exhale. In time, and with practice, you may even begin to feel like a balloon—buoyant, light as air. Feeling light.

It's normal to feel heavy, even rooted, at the beginning of this exercise; it's a pleasant, relaxed state you'll want to maintain for a long while. This temporary heavy feeling is the chi flowing and balancing all the yin and yang energies throughout your body. Don't be surprised if you emerge from Universal Life Post feeling anything but leaden—feeling full of energy, free of the feelings or thoughts that might have weighted you down. Standing meditation is a means of harvesting internal energy, storing it in the tan tien, and making it available for healing and/or defense.

HEAVEN/MAN-WOMAN/EARTH

According to chi philosophy, there is movement in stillness, and stillness in movement. Whereas Universal Life Post belongs in the family of "static" chi gong exercises, there are many dynamic forms as well: Heaven/Man-Woman/Earth illustrates one that can be likened to the growth of a tree, rooted in earth but reaching heavenward.

Stand erect and allow yourself to relax for several minutes, as we've discussed. Then adjust your stance so that your feet are spread apart and each foot points out at a 45-

degree angle. Flex your toes and lightly grab the ground with them as if they were claws—or roots. The sole of your foot should be slightly arched. Imagine yourself not simplying standing on the earth, but growing out from it, absorbing its energies as a tree would soak up water and nutrients from the soil.

Now slowly bend your knees until your kneecaps are out over your toes. As you're descending, bring your hands together, back to back, fingertips pointing earthward. Lower yourself as far as you can do so comfortably, keeping your back straight and your hands together. As you lower yourself, try and coordinate your breathing so that you're inhaling for the length of the downward journey. Remember to "belly breathe," so that your abdomen, not your chest, goes in and out (Figures 5, 6, 7, 8).

When you've filled your lungs and feel the need to exhale, relax the soles of your feet and slowly begin to rise. Again, the idea is to coordinate your breath with your movement, exhaling as you rise. Gradually straighten your knees, lift your hands, open your hands outward to the sky, reach up your arms, arch your back, and extend your arms backward as far as you're able, all to the tempo of letting out your breath. You should feel your joints open, your muscles stretch. Imagine you're a tree and you can feel the sap running, the chi flowing. Imagine your arms are branches and your fingertips are leaves, stretching above the forest canopy to absorb the sun's rays. Your feet remain rooted. Your spine is as strong and flexible as a tree trunk. You're a living link between earth and sky, a conduit for the energy that remains constant but everchanging in the universe (Figures 9, 10, 11, 12, 13, 14, 15).

Now it's time to repeat the motion. Relax your arms, start to inhale, and sink as you did before, bringing your hands together with fingers pointed down. Repeat this whole cycle of sinking and rising, inhaling and exhaling,

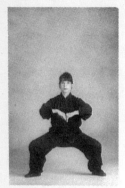

FIGURE 5

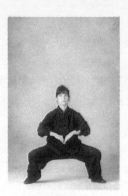

FIGURE 6

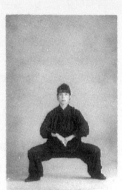

FIGURE 7

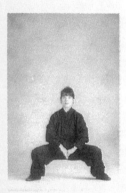

FIGURE 8

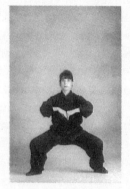

FIGURE 9

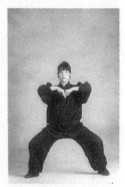

FIGURE 10

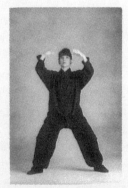

FIGURE 11

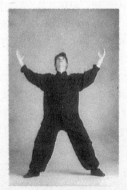

FIGURE 12

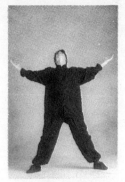

FIGURE 13

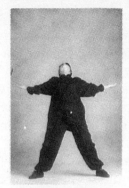

FIGURE 14

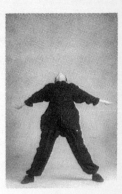

FIGURE 15

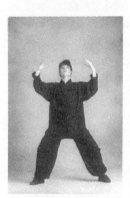

FIGURE 16

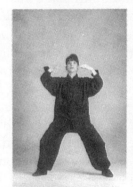

FIGURE 17

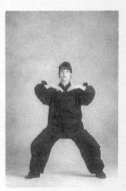

FIGURE 18

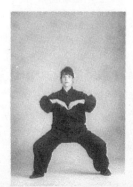

FIGURE 19

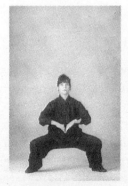

FIGURE 20

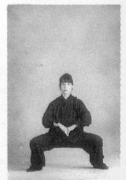

FIGURE 21

ten times. Don't worry if you pause between cycles and take a breath or two: the important thing is to breathe in while you're dropping and breathe out while you're rising. Work toward drawing one long, deep breath while you're bending your knees and sinking earthward; practice letting out that breath slowly enough so that you're embracing the sky just as you feel the need to inhale again (Figures 16, 17, 18, 19, 20, 21).

At first, you may not be able to do ten cycles; start with fewer repetitions, until you feel comfortable with the movement. Within a week you'll find that your range of motion and your endurance have increased. In fact, just as a tree grows, increasing the size and length of its roots, absorbing life-giving energy from both sun and soil, strengthening its trunk while extending its branches—so too will you grow. Gradually you'll tone your legs, back, and arms. You'll find yourself more flexible and free of pain in your upper back, shoulders, and knees. You'll feel more energized, thanks to increased blood flow and lung capacity. You'll be centered. Balanced. As durable as an oak, as yielding as a willow. You'll complete the circuit of energy between atmosphere and earth. Like a tree, you will have transmuted sunlight, oxygen, water, and nutrients into life itself.

TAI CHI EXERCISE FOR LONG LIFE

Throughout this book we have emphasized the importance of unity and harmony: how mental, physical, and spiritual health are interrelated, imbalance in one sphere affecting the balance and harmony of the whole. This is by no means a new idea. The Chinese have embraced this holistic phi- losophy and incorporated it into their art, their science, and their religion for millennia. There is no separation, in fact, between disciplines as seemingly unrelated as, say, herbology and Tai Chi: underlying both is the concept of nurturing or restoring chi so that all life systems may work harmoniously, counterbalancing each other much as yin and yang oppose each other in the Chinese symbol we introduced you to earlier.

Tai Chi—particularly the exercise we're going to show you now—is emblematic of that belief: when performed correctly, the movements flow so seamlessly together that it's hard to distinguish the beginning or end of one cycle. Practicing Tai Chi so that the chi will flow is often compared to unwinding silk from a cocoon so that the thread doesn't break: a steady, even motion is the secret. If you can master that steady flow of mind and body united in purpose, then health and long life will be yours.

The Long Life exercise is literally circular. A circle illustrates both infinite motion and conservation of energy. A circle traces the route of all life energy, from birth, to death, to decay and the nourishment of new life. A circle embodies the circuit of blood and oxygen in the human body; a rising circle, or spiral, describes the path of our emotional development and spiritual enlightenment. In this exercise, an imaginary circle will guide both the motion of your limbs and the direction of your thoughts.

To begin, stand so that your chin is tilted slightly downward, hiding your throat; your nose will come into line with your navel. Consciously relax your neck and shoulders. It may help to imagine that your head is suspended from above, anchored to the sky or ceiling with a thread that's attached to your crown. If you can allow your head to hang suspended, neck and shoulders will naturally fall away, opening up your spinal column for blood and chi to circulate. Your shoulders will be slightly forward, your spine will be straight. Your hands should be open, and naturally flexed.

Gaze forward, but don't fix on anything; rather, relax your focus, concentrating instead on your posture and the open passageways you've created by standing erect and relaxed.

Breathe in and out slowly through your nose. This will be easier if you allow your tongue to rest lightly against the roof of your mouth. Keep your mouth closed.

If you tilt your pelvis slightly forward and upward, your tailbone will sink and you will be utterly centered, ready to move in any direction without fear of losing your balance. Don't lock your knees; relax your hips. You shouldn't feel any strain. Continue breathing, allowing your abdomen to expand and deflate. From this posture, all Tai Chi begins.

Now place one foot in front of the other—say, right in front of left—right heel to left toes. To maintain this stance you'll find your left knee bending slightly.

Position your hands in front of you at waist height as though you were holding a volleyball (Figure 22). You're

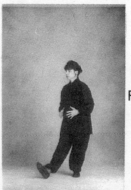

FIGURE 22

going to move this imaginary ball through space, tracing an imaginary circle out in front of you—as if you were rolling that ball around the rim of a big marching-band drum sticking out from your chest. The challenge is to move the ball around and around, rocking forward onto your toes and then back onto your heels, all the while *keeping your body at the same height.*

Okay. Start by moving the ball up and forward, as though over the top of the drum (Figures 23, 24, 25). Shift your weight forward so that you can push the ball out as far as possible without letting go (Figure 26). Bring the ball back toward you, along the lower rim of the invisible drum (Figure 27). You'll now be shifting your weight back on your heels as you bring the ball closer (Figure 28). Go as far back on your heels as you can in order to get the ball up between your waist and the drum (Figure 29). When you've reached this point and you're starting to shift forward to push the ball up and over the top again, you've completed one cycle (Figure 30).

Repeat this circling motion for two to five minutes, then stop, switch the placement of your feet—left in front of right, now—and do two to five minutes of circling on that side as well.

When you've got the movement down so that you don't have to think about it, try coordinating your breathing: inhale as the ball approaches you, exhale as you push the ball away. Remember to breathe in and out through your nose and to allow your abdomen, not your chest, to do the expanding and contracting. You'll find that you'll need to slow down the pace at which you direct the ball around the drum in order to coordinate your breathing with your movement.

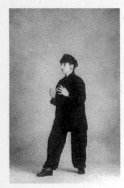

FIGURE 23

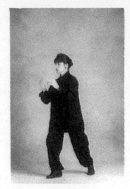

FIGURE 24

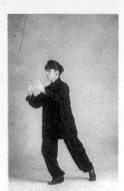

FIGURE 25

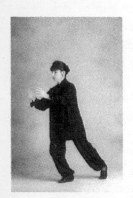

FIGURE 26

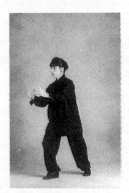

FIGURE 27

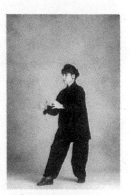

FIGURE 28

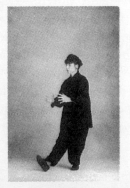

FIGURE 29

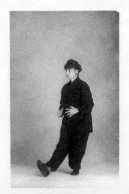

FIGURE 30

CAN YOU FEEL YOUR CHI?

Like anything else worth doing, Tai Chi pays out more benefits the more time you invest in perfecting it. First, you've got to learn the moves. When you've got them down pat, when they flow as if you were "swimming in air," you can incorporate your breathing so that it both follows and directs your movements. In time, through many repetitions, you will enjoy the meditative aspect of your motion. And in time, through many repetitions, you may be surprised to feel something quite physical: a warmth, a tingling, a fluidity, an elation, a flush of well-being. That's *chi*! And it's what you've been cultivating by doing these Tai Chi and chi gong exercises.

Don't think of moving your chi as a goal. Don't think of it as some mystical, transcendent thing you'll never experience. Don't believe you even have to believe in it! Tai Chi and chi gong, like every other "tool" we've provided you with in this book, work best when you allow them to work by just doing them. We want you literally "to go through the motions." It's entirely natural to take up the practice of Tai Chi really wanting to feel this elusive chi, then feeling vaguely disappointed when you don't feel anything, and then despairing that you ever will. Don't allow yourself to be defeated by your own thoughts. Repeat the exercises, if for no other reason than you'll feel physically energized, more limber, more balanced. Focus on your tan tien. Suspend disbelief. And know that through this practice, by increasing your blood flow, by moving and breathing, health, balance, and optimal weight loss are all achievable.

Getting It All Together

Your Game Plan for Health

"*If I did all I'm supposed to do for Feeling Light,*" one of our participants told us, "*I'd never get out the door each day. I'm lucky if I get done half of what I've got to do as it is.*"

"*I'm under a lot of stress right now,*" another client insisted, "*so I've just not been able to do the vitamins and herbs and everything.*"

And finally: "*I just don't have the time for this.*"

Let us reassure you that you do, indeed, have the time. Beginning today, you have the rest of your life. By baby steps, and then by leaps and bounds, you will adopt components of Feeling Light until it's no longer a program—it's your life.

Unlike any weight management program you've ever been on (and then off), there's no clock you've got to beat, no goal you've got to meet, no weight you've got to attain by next week *or else*. Feeling Light is a conversation you have with yourself, not some sort of judgmental keep-with-the-group thing. Every aspect of Feeling Light that you incorporate, however haltingly, advances your health and puts you one step away from a weight problem. When you make excuses, you simply delay your own journey.

Stress is one of the least valid reasons for putting the program on hold. We're all living with a lot of stress, and the more we feel it, the more imperative it is that we employ the tools Feeling Light gives us to combat it. As our client Lynn has already noted, stress may be *the result* of not taking the supplements, of eating a lot of meat and dairy, of failing to take time out for breathing, exercising, and reflection.

Feeling Light is a blueprint for a new way of life, one that makes no room for weight problems. But remember that this house will start rather modestly, from the ground up. We've given you the foundation, and all the tools and building materials you'll need; now we'll tell you how to frame it out, day by day, week by week, month after month, season after season. Before you know it, you'll be moving into your dream house.

A FEELING LIGHT DAY

> Every day, try and employ these basic tools:
>
> • the Smoothie
> • daily affirmations
> • breathing exercises
> • stretching
> • Tai Chi
> • meditation
> • self acupressure
> • flower essences
> • rebounding or other exercise

Understand that there will be days when you use all of them, days when you rely on four or five, and days where you're lucky to pick up one of them. No one is foreman on this job, overseeing your labors: it's just you, and it's your house. The more tools you use, the more efficient you'll be. There are good days, better days, and best days.

Here's how one of your best days might look:

Upon waking, **breathe**. Stand up straight, and practice your chi gong breathing exercises (see Chapter 11) for five to ten minutes, right there in your bedroom.

Now **stretch** as we described in Chapter 3. **Recite** your **daily affirmations** as you stretch. Move to a bigger room, or go outside, and do repetitions of Tai Chi for ten minutes.

Shower "mindfully," **as a meditative ritual**—see Chapter 2.

Prepare and **drink the Feeling Light Smoothie**. (That

makes four components of the program you've worked in, and it's only breakfast!)

If out of habit or craving or rebellion you feel tempted to snack midmorning, **massage the ear pressure points** we detail in Chapter 10. **Recite** your **daily affirmations**. **Take several deep, cleansing breaths**. **Sip** from a large cup of water prepared with all five **flower essences.**

For lunch, **eat according to the healthy food guidelines** we outlined in Chapter 6; see our menu selections (below); or **adopt a mono-food cleansing fast**—brown rice, or watermelon, or apple juice. For a refresher on cleansing methods, see Chapter 5.

At workday's end, **substitute a vigorous walk or five minutes of rebounding** for that cocktail or snack you normally rely on as a transition into leisure time. Make your exercise mindful, or **meditate for ten minutes** in a quiet place.

Dinner, like lunch, **should adhere to Feeling Light guidelines**—remember, no more than three animal-protein meals per week. Or, continue with the mono-food or juice fast. Again, to fend off cravings for sweets or bedtime snacks, **practice acupressure, breathe deeply, and sip from the flower essence drink**. Before retiring for the evening, **recite again the daily affirmations**.

Congratulations: you've used every tool in the Feeling Light kit. Your house is taking shape!

A MONTHLY PLANNER

Not everyone, of course, can read a blueprint and know just how to get started. For most of us, in fact, there's a warm-up, get-acquainted, trial-and-error learning period that necessarily precedes actual construction. That period

can take weeks. Here's how we recommend you work up
to the job.

Week One
- Begin a slow detox, using dandelion, milk thistle, and
  burdock root.
- Begin taking the Feeling Light Smoothie.
- Practice your breathing, stretching, and Tai Chi exer-
  cises.
- Massage ear acupressure points to stave off cravings.
- Make one day a week (Monday seems to be ideal) a
  mono-food fast—brown rice, or a fruit, or a juice only.

Week Two
  In addition to the above:
- Walk. Whether your tolerance is five minutes or thirty,
  something is better than nothing. Do what you can.
- Get a rebounder, or mini-trampoline, and jump for two
  to five minutes.
- Mix up a large water bottle or thermos with the flower
  essences and sip from it all day.
- Set aside ten minutes daily for practicing meditation.
- Practice Tai Chi for five to ten minutes.

Week Three
  In addition to all of the above:
- Begin to incorporate nutritional supplements that aid
  in fat metabolism and help eliminate cravings.
- Choose herbs or a formulation that will address your
  needs.
- Increase rebounding to five or seven minutes daily.
- Begin each day with breathing, Tai Chi, daily affir-
  mations, and the Smoothie.
- End each day with a recitation of the affirmations.

Week Four
  Now you are ready to incorporate:
- A longer fast. See the Seasonal Chart for suggestions.

Remind yourself that you can always stop. It's easier than you think!

DESIGNING A BALANCED MEAL

If you lived through the last vegetarian trend, you may remember the concern about "complete proteins." Twenty some years ago, nutritionists were of a mind that unless you combined your legumes and grains correctly, your body would not be fueled with the raw materials necessary to manufacture essential proteins.

Extensive research has debunked this notion. The fact is, it's virtually impossible to *not* get enough protein, even on a strict no-meat, no-dairy diet—regardless of food combinations. If no more than five percent of our daily calories should come from protein, as the World Health Organization indicates, then if anything, our concern should be in designing meals that cut way back on this particular fuel.

The reason, as we've already spelled out in previous chapters, is that protein foods are acidifying when metabolized. We're not talking about the alkalinity or acidity of the food itself, nor of the effect the food has on the pH of your stomach (although protein can affect stomach acidity): we're talking about the effect of these foods on your blood pH, which cannot deviate much from neutral without severe consequences—coma, convulsions, even death. To keep blood pH balanced and neutral, your body will 1) buffer acidity with calcium leached from its bone stores; 2) reduce acids into water and carbon dioxide for elimination via the kidneys and lungs; 3) reroute the acids back into the stomach; 4) store them as mineral salts. When acid is a constant presence, your body begins to suffer the effects of constantly managing it. Osteoporosis, nervous disorders, chronic fatigue, kidney stones, kidney damage, gallstones, bone spurs, cataracts, arthritis, gout, and an impaired immune system all are conditions associated with acidosis, or excessive blood acidity.

But you don't need to be a chemist to keep your meals balanced. Pictured here is the yin/yang food gradient we discussed in Chapter 4. It just so happens that foods classified as **yin** by and large have an **alkalizing** effect on blood pH, and foods classified as **yang**, an **acidifying** effect. Foods in the middle are neutral, meaning they don't affect blood pH either way. Balance, as would appear obvious by the chart we offer on the next page, lies in complementing yin foods with yang, or eating neutral or nearly-neutral foods such as brown rice.

The Chinese balanced their intake of yin and yang foods according to season, tempering summer's abundance of raw fruits and squashes with winter's cornucopia of cooked root vegetables. Today, of course, supermarkets, refrigeration, and long-distance shipping have obliterated the notion of season, but that means simply that in the course of any given day, you should strive to balance raw foods with cooked, fruits with vegetables, beans with rice, wine with meat, and so on. Use very sparingly or not at all foods that lie at the extremes.

A WEEK AT A GLANCE

We encourage our clients to make up their own menus, following the basic guidelines we established in Chapter 6. One reason: formulaic weekly menus smack of diets, or regimens where deviation spells failure—and that just isn't what Feeling Light is about. Also, from experience we've noted that most people do better when they're allowed to reinvent their meals at their own pace. (Dictating what you should eat can have a slingshot effect: you follow our every

YIN ← COOLING **WARMING → YANG**

Derivatives	Fruits	Vegetables	Light Grains	Brown Rice	Grains	Nuts & Legumes	Fish & Fowl	Meats & Eggs
extremely yin	very yin	yin	slightly yin	NEUTRAL	slightly yang	yang	very yang	extremely yang
drugs	tropical fruit	bean sprouts	millet		bulgur	nuts	cooked fish	beef
artificial sweeteners	fresh fruit	leafy vegetables	corn		oats	legumes (lentils, beans)	shellfish	pork
table salt	potato	cruciferous vegetables	white basmati		buckwheat	seeds	turkey	lamb
preservatives	tomato	summer squashes	barley wheat		amaranth	winter squashes	chicken	game
	peppers	salad greens	quinoa		spelt	root vegetables	cheese	organ meats
	eggplant	seaweeds						eggs
	milk	soybean curd (tofu)						sugars
		dried fruit						
		raw fish						
		yogurt						

Most Yin   Most Yang

suggestion for every meal for a week or two, and then you revert back to all your old ways.)

That being said, we also acknowledge that when you're new to something, it's hard to be creative: you want direction, plus a little nudge to give you momentum. Hence we've created menus here to give you ideas, to give you a model of better eating. If you're inspired to follow our suggestions to the letter, good for you—but bear in mind that relearning food selection, preparation, and meal planning is a process, one that rarely supplants in a few short weeks years of shopping and cooking as an omnivore. Our attitudes toward food may change overnight, but our ability to actually put into practice our good instincts can take time.

A word on eating a la Feeling Light: **Make portions small**. If you finish the meal and feel truly hungry, you can always put more on your plate, but you may surprise yourself by finding that you're not as hungry as habit dictates. That's why it's also absolutely critical that you **learn to eat slowly.** Between bites, put your fork down. You'll feel fuller faster; you won't smother the little voice that's telling you when you've had enough to meet your needs. For that matter, you don't need to eat everything we suggest for a meal. If you're full before you've had the fruit for dessert, by all means, STOP.

—Spring/Summer Menus—

MONDAY

Breakfast: Mix up our Smoothie or fix a bowl of your favorite fresh fruit. Alternatively, try puffed rice or wheat with soy or rice milk (a heckuva lot creamier than skim milk, and tastier, too). Slice some apricots, or rehydrate with a glass of 100 percent juice. Instead of coffee, try Roma, Cafix, Pero, or any of our other suggestions in Chapter Six, including herbal teas. Or dissolve a packet of instant miso in hot water. If you use the paste, use just a teaspoon per cup.

Lunch: Basmati white rice topped with tofu sesame saute.

It's a cinch: while the rice is cooking, saute half a cup of onions and two or three cloves of garlic with half a teaspoon of olive oil. Slice a brick of firm tofu into quarter-inch-thick rectangles and throw them into the skillet, turning them gently until they're browned on both sides. Dash two drops of tamari on each side and pan-fry for a few seconds; smother with sesame seeds, turn gently, and fry for a moment. Smother remaining side with seeds, and transfer slices to a Pyrex baking dish. Bake covered for 5–7 minutes at 275 degrees. A bowl of cold gazpacho with a dollop of nonfat plain yogurt—dairy should be used as a condiment only.

Dinner: Dark-leaved salad greens (no iceberg, please) with olive oil and vinegar. Experiment with different flavored vinegars! Top angel hair pasta with cooked plum tomatoes and oregano. Stir-fry snow peas, carrots, and broccoli.

TUESDAY

Breakfast: Okay, you know the drill: Smoothie or fresh fruit. Or, one poached egg on a slice of whole wheat bread, one-quarter cantaloupe (or juice), and an herbal tea or grain beverage/coffee substitute.

Lunch: Salad of sliced tomatoes with basil and oregano, and a tofu burger. Pretty hippie, huh? You'll love it. For dessert, quarter a mango.

Dinner: Basmati white rice; steamed yellow crooked squash and zucchini (a little lemon pepper perks it up); baked chicken breast (no skin, please) with sweet 'n' sour sauce—and we don't mean that sticky orange stuff. Here's the sauce:

    2 tsps rice vinegar
    2 tbs tamari
    1/4 cup tomato paste plus 1 tsp maple syrup
    2 tsps ginger
    2 cloves garlic, minced
    1/3 cup chicken broth or water
    1 tsp kudzu (the powdered root of an herb used in place of cornstarch as a thickener)

Combine it all in a saucepan and cook over medium heat, stirring constantly, until the mixture simmers and thickens. Cool. Marinate chicken or tofu in it for 2 hours, or in the fridge overnight.

For dessert, fix a fruit salad.

WEDNESDAY

Breakfast: Smoothie or fruit or: Shredded Wheat or Grape Nuts with soy or rice milk (you can do it); one cup of strawberries and bananas; and herbal tea, miso cup, or a grain beverage.

Lunch: Tuna (yes, it's in a can, but we're realistic) on a bed of arugula and romaine leaves with tomatoes and balsamic vinegar dressing. Once you substitute balsamic vinegar for the plain ol' stuff, you won't want to go back.

Combine:
    1/4 tsp pepper
    1 tbs cold-pressed extra-virgin olive oil
    1 tbs balsamic vinegar
    1/4 tsp dry mustard

In a small bowl and beat until smooth with a fork. Add 2 more tablespoons olive oil, whisk again; add 1 tablespoon balsamic vinegar, 3 more tablespoons olive oil, and whisk again; season with 2 cloves of minced garlic, dillweed, basil, and oregano, and shake well. To die for—on salads, veggies, and grains. We're especially fond of this dressing on "mesculin greens"—the mix of arugula, radicchio, dandelion, and other specialty lettuces now carried in many supermarkets as well as health food and Asian produce markets.

Flesh out the meal with brown rice and a fruit salad.

Dinner: Boston bibb lettuce with sun-dried tomatoes and sesame-poppyseed dressing. You can make this in a snap—much tastier than anything you can buy prepared.

2/3 cup pineapple juice
1 tsp grated fresh ginger
1 tbs mirin (a sweetened sake sold in health
    food stores or Asian markets)
1/4 tsp sesame oil
1 tbs sesame seeds, toasted
1 tbs poppy seeds
3 tbs nonfat plain yogurt

Blend all ingredients in a blender, or whisk well.

Then: shiitake mushrooms sauteed with slivered carrots and onions; half a baked potato; and—are you ready for this? Miso tofu soup. Pretty soon you'll be wearing bell bottoms and love beads. Here's how to make it:

2 carrots sliced into coins
1/2 onion, sliced
4 cups water
brick of firm tofu, cubed

Combine in saucepan, bring to boil, simmer for 20 minutes. Remove from heat. Put 2 big tablespoons (more or less to taste) of miso paste—red, black, white, tan, it doesn't matter what variety—in a bowl, add some of the soup broth, and stir into a paste before adding it back to the soup. Optional: Before cooking the soup, add two pieces of kombu seaweed that have been soaked for 20 minutes, and/or 2 tablespoons of adzuki beans that have been soaked overnight.

THURSDAY
Breakfast: Smoothie, or just fruit, or: One cup yogurt (if it's nonfat, with no added sugar, yogurt

is the permissible dairy exception because of its healthful acidophilus content); sliced bananas or other fruit (added to yogurt, or by itself); half a whole-grain bagel; and the usual non-coffee beverage options.

Lunch: White basmati rice; steamed broccoli, cauliflower, and carrots sprinkled with sesame seeds; and two Medjool dates. If you've never experienced these monster dates, you're in for a real treat. They make caramels look dietetic.

Dinner: Endive/radicchio/romaine salad with sesame-poppyseed dressing; vidalia onions (they're as sweet as apples), red peppers, portobello mushroom slices, and zucchini halves dabbed in barbecue sauce and grilled; roasted corn-on-the-cob (leave the husks on and turn on the grill for 20 minutes til husks are blackened); and baked beans. No dessert—the beans have enough brown sugar to be a treat!

FRIDAY
Breakfast: Smoothie or fruit or: Cream of Wheat with soy or rice milk (admit it—it's growing on you); juice, or a cup of blueberries/raspberries/strawberries; and hot herbal or grain beverage.

Lunch: Spinach salad with mushrooms, mandarin oranges, and oil and balsamic vinegar dressing; half a turkey sandwich on whole wheat bread with lettuce and tomato but absolutely no mayo, not even that tasteless goop they call "fat-free"; and a sliced apple.

Dinner: Brown rice primavera (cauliflower, broccoli, carrots); onion soup, minus the bread blobs and that roof of melted cheese you may be used to; salad of red leaf lettuce, red grapes, sunflower seeds, and Miso French dressing. For the dressing—which is just as good on pasta, or on vegetables:

> 1 tsp honey mustard
> 2 tbs minced garlic
> 1/4 cup apple cider
> juice of a whole lemon
> 1 tbs extra virgin olive oil
> 3 tbs fresh tomato puree or juice
> 1 tsp miso paste
> a pinch of cayenne or paprika for zest
>   (optional)

For dessert, treat yourself to a half cup of mango sorbet. If you want to experience something divine, try mixing the sorbet with vanilla frozen yogurt. Häagen-Dazs makes both, without additives or derivatives. Yum!

SATURDAY
Breakfast: Smoothie or fruit or: Toasted oat bran English muffin with a teaspoon of sesame butter (tahini) and all-fruit/sugarless jam; fruit salad. Once you're in balance and eating to maintain it, you can introduce very small amounts of butter. (Use clarified butter, which is made by melting the butter over very low heat until the oils and milk solids separate; discard the milk solids.) But you may no longer feel the need, especially if you experiment with some of the fruit and nut butters.

Lunch: A half cup of carrot/celery juice; tri-color pasta and sauteed vegetable salad; half a whole wheat bagel with all-fruit/sugarless jam.

Dinner: Large tossed salad; spinach spaghetti pasta with turkey meatballs and tomato sauce (process fresh tomatoes for a chunky, tangy sauce seasoned with fresh basil and oregano); steamed broccoli; and melon ball fruit salad.

SUNDAY
Breakfast: Smoothie or fruit or: One scrambled egg; one whole grain waffle with a teaspoon of real maple syrup (you'll wonder how you tolerated that corn syrup product for so long); and sliced peaches.

Lunch: Brown rice with sesame seeds and teriyaki sauce; lentil soup; and tossed salad with Green Goddess dressing:

> 8 oz soft or silken tofu, mashed
> 1 tsp dijon mustard
> 2 tbs chopped cilantro
> 1 whole scallion, chopped fine
> 1 tbs lemon juice
> 1 tbs rice vinegar
> 1 tbs mirin
> 2 small cloves garlic, chopped
> splash of tamari
> dash of pepper
> 1 tsp capers
> 1/4-1/2 cup water as needed for consistency

Process in food processor till creamy.

Dinner: Baked lemon garlic flounder; cooked millet (it sure beats Minute Rice) mixed with sauteed onions; string beans, baby carrots, and sliced portobello mushrooms sauteed with garlic and onions; and half a grapefruit (why just for breakfast?).

Remember: One day each week—preferably, the same day—consume only apple juice, or brown rice and spring water, for a cleansing fast.

—FALL/WINTER MENUS—

MONDAY
Breakfast: Smoothie or fruit or: Oatmeal sprinkled with flax seeds, with soy or rice milk; half a grapefruit; herbal or grain beverages.

Lunch: Vegetable soup; pita bread stuffed with hummus, celery, cucumber, and black olives; applesauce. Homemade is best: Add a little water to apple slices and simmer until they're very soft. Process in a food processor if you like it smooth.

Dinner: Baked red snapper; steamed or roasted sweet potato (you won't even need butter or toppings, it's so sweet); and baked spaghetti squash with garlic and tamari. To fix the squash—that big yellow thing you've always wondered what to do with—halve it, scoop out and discard the seeds, and put it in a baking dish with a little water in the dish. Smear insides of squash with a teaspoon of this mixture:

> **3 garlic cloves, minced**
> **1/2 cup extra-virgin olive oil**
> **1/2 tsp to 1 tsp tamari**

Bake at 350 degrees for 40 minutes, or until tender. The garlic/tamari sauce is great on vegetables, grains, and pastas—but use it very sparingly.

TUESDAY
Breakfast: Smoothie or fruit or hot nine-grain cereal with soy or rice milk; stewed prunes; herbal or grain beverage.

Lunch: Black bean soup; whole wheat pita bread stuffed with tomatoes, soy cheese (another wondrous alternative to dairy), and sprouts (alfalfa or radish or mung bean—they're not just fodder for flower children); and baked pear sprinkled with granola.

Dinner: Romaine, shredded red cabbage, diced red peppers, and tomato salad with lemon dijon dressing; linguine with pignole nuts (2 tablespoons, max) and garlic/tamari dressing; broccoli rabe; and—brace yourself—tempeh saute. Yep—another weird soybean dish. Tempeh looks like a paper pulp product, but wait till you try it: Cut the slab into cubes and saute it with garlic and onion until it's toasted and crunchy. Just before serving, add a dash of tamari and toss. Yum!

As for the lemon dijon dressing, whisk together:

1/4 cup balsamic vinegar
1/4 cup water
1 tsp lemon juice
1/4 cup oil
3 tsp tamari
4 cloves minced garlic
1 tsp prepared dijon mustard

This dressing is marvelous on rice, pasta, or vegetables, too.

WEDNESDAY
Breakfast: Smoothie or fruit or: Hot brown rice with soy milk, cinnamon, and honey or maple syrup; carrot or apple juice; hot herbal or grain beverage.

Lunch: Pea soup (no ham, no ham bone, just the humble pea); small cabbage salad; one slice toasted whole wheat bread, smeared with 1 teaspoon tahini.

Dinner: Tofu burger or tofu dog (can you believe we haven't exhausted these darn soybean spinoffs yet?); roasted red potatoes with garlic (toss cubed potatoes with coarse sea salt, minced fresh garlic, a splash of balsamic vinegar, and crumbled rosemary before baking uncovered at 400 degrees); steamed Swiss chard with mushrooms and green onions; sliced bananas and kiwifruit.

THURSDAY
Breakfast: Smoothie or fruit or: Wheatena with soy or rice milk; a tangerine; and herbal or grain beverage.

Lunch: Cabbage soup (don't cook it to death, or the cabbage gets slimy); fruit salad; and a slice of whole grain bread. If it's a really good bread, you won't miss the spread. Some of the bread-in-a-bag mixes are great; use seltzer for the liquid. Your friends will be wowed.

Dinner: Spinach and mushroom casserole; lima beans with fennel seeds and lemon juice; small tossed salad with orange-ginger dressing.

Process till smooth:
   3 tsp tahini
   2 tsp balsamic vinegar
   1/2 cup vegetable stock
   1 medium orange, sectioned and seeded
   1 tsp honey mustard
   1 tsp grated fresh ginger
   pinch of black peppers

FRIDAY
Breakfast: Smoothie or fruit or: Oatmeal with soy or rice milk; sliced bananas (in or out of the oatmeal); and a cup of miso.

Lunch: Spinach, beet, mushroom, and scallion salad with lemon-dijon dressing; minestrone soup; and baked apple.

Dinner: Tofu dogs and sauerkraut (try and avoid the canned stuff; it's easy to make your own); roasted carrots, parsnips, and beets; and baked apple. (We're exploiting the harvest; apples that have been in cold storage for untold weeks just don't compare. Experiment with different varieties—you don't have to stick with McIntosh.)

SATURDAY
Breakfast: Smoothie or fruit or: Grape Nuts with soy or rice milk (now you've got your friends trying it); sliced pear (not canned, please); and herbal or grain beverage.

Lunch: Small tossed salad with dijon/garlic dressing; corn chowder; half a turkey sandwich with cranberry sauce (canned is okay, but fresh will knock your socks off, especially if it's made with ginger) on whole wheat bread.

Dinner: Sweet potato/carrot soup (super carotene concoction!); sauteed asparagus and onions with lemon wedges; vegetarian chili over couscous. Very fortifying.

SUNDAY
Breakfast: Smoothie or fruit or: Eggwhite omelette with green peppers and onions; stewed prunes; and herbal or grain beverage.

Lunch: Cucumber and fresh dill salad; steamed artichoke; brown rice with garlic/tamari dressing.

Dinner: Small romaine salad with marinated artichoke hearts, cherry tomatoes, and balsamic vinaigrette; tempeh with sweet 'n' sour sauce (our own; see above); ziti baked with broccoli.

Remember: One day each week—preferably, the same day—consume only apple juice, or brown rice and spring water, for a cleansing fast.

A PLAN FOR ALL SEASONS

Put it all together—the days, the weeks, the months—and here's what Feeling Light looks like over a year's time: A balance of summer fasting and winter nourishing, spring cleaning and fall preparation.

Spring

Herbs
> dandelion
> milk thistle
> burdock
> yellow dock

Foods
> lightly steamed vegetables
> light grains (barley, quinoa)
> adzuki beans
> light soups or broths
> room-temperature drinks
> cup of miso

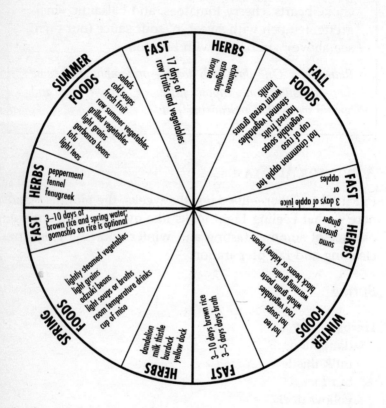

SUMMER

FOODS
salads
cold soups
fresh fruit
raw summer vegetables
grilled vegetables
light grains
garbanzo beans
tofu
light teas

FAST
17 days of
raw fruits and vegetables

HERBS
echinacea
astragalus
licorice

FALL

FOODS
lentils
warm cereal grains
steamed vegetables
harvest fruits
cup of miso
hot cinnamon apple tea

FAST
3 days of apple juice
or
apples

HERBS
peppermint
fennel
fenugreek

HERBS
suma
ginseng
ginger

FAST
3–10 days of
brown rice and spring water;
gomashio on rice is optional

FOODS
lightly steamed vegetables
light grains
adzuki beans
light soups or broths
room temperature drinks
cup of miso

WINTER

FOODS
hot tea
hot soups
root vegetables
whole grain pasta
warming grains
black beans or kidney beans

SPRING

HERBS
dandelion
milk thistle
burdock
yellow dock

FAST
3–10 days brown rice
3–5 days days broth

FEELING LIGHT THROUGH THE CHANGE OF SEASONS.

Fast
> 3–10 days of brown rice and spring water; gomashio
> on rice is optional

Summer

Herbs
> peppermint
> fennel
> fenugreek

Foods
> salads
> cold soups
> fresh fruit
> raw summer vegetables (tomatoes, cucumbers, yellow
> squash, zucchini)
> grilled vegetables (onions, peppers, eggplant, zucchini)
> light grains (millet, white basmati rice, couscous, qui-
> noa, corn)
> garbanzo beans
> tofu
> light teas (hibiscus coolers)
> cool drinks

Fast
> 17 days of raw fruits and vegetables

Fall

Herbs
> echinacea
> astragalus
> licorice

Foods

> vegetable soups
> harvest fruits (apples, pears)
> steamed vegetables
> warm cereal grains (oats, amaranth)
> lentils
> hot apple-cinnamon tea
> cup of miso

Fast

> 3 days of apples or apple juice

Winter

Herbs

> suma
> ginseng
> ginger

Foods

> hot soups
> root vegetables (potatoes, turnips, carrots, parsnips)
> whole grain pastas
> warming grains (bulgur, buckwheat, brown rice, spelt)
> black beans or kidney beans
> hot tea

Fast

> 3–10 days of brown rice
> or 3–5 days of vegetable broth

THE BIG PICTURE

All of life is cyclical.

Each day, each month, each season, each year, each lifetime has its ebbs and tides. Every life process, every observed phenomenon embraces the polarities of light and dark, growth and recession, push and pull, positive and negative.

These mutually defining yin and yang forces, dueling eternally for dominance, describe balance in the individual as well as balance in the cosmos. There is an ebb and tide to our appetites, according to excess and deficiency within. Our needs—mentally, physiologically, and spiritually— are constantly changing. Provided we're tuned to those needs, and provided we heed their signals, we can maintain balance, health, and optimal weight despite our state of flux.

Feeling Light is above all a program designed to restore that dynamic equilibrium; it works with your natural cycling, not in defiance of it. It forgives periods of weakness; it exploits periods of strength. It allows for holidays, dinners out, glasses of wine, and the occasional binge; it acknowledges that you live with stress, pollution, frozen vegetables, and finicky family members. It does not berate you for your imperfections; it urges you to reach for your full potential.

Practiced daily, practiced weekly, practiced seasonally, Feeling Light is going to strip off those protective layers of fat so that you may emerge as newly born and beautiful as a butterfly emerges from its chrysalis. You'll have shed those heavy, smothering, deadening layers for a streamlined body that revels in its energy. You will feel light; you will be lighter, whether you measure your progress in pounds or inches, mood or energy levels, skin elasticity or muscle tone, or even visits to the doctor.

You have it within you to achieve this evolution. And you have in your hands all the guidance you need. It's never too late. Today can be a good day. Tomorrow can be a better day.

The best days of all lie just ahead.

APPENDIX

Resources

FINDING THE RIGHT HEALTH PRACTITIONER

National Commission for the Certification of
  Acupuncturists
1424 16th Street NW, Suite 501
Washington, District of Columbia 20036
(202) 232-1404

American Association of Naturopathic Physicians
2366 Eastlake Avenue East, Suite 322
P.O. Box 20386
Seattle, Washington 98102
(206) 323-7610

American Holistic Medical Association
4101 Lake Boone Trail, Suite 201
Raleigh, North Carolina 27607
(919) 787-5146

National Center for Homeopathy
801 North Fairfax Street
Alexandria, Virginia 22314
(703) 548-7790

LEARN MORE ABOUT FLOWER ESSENCES

Bach, Edward, M.D. and F.J. Wheeler. The Bach Flower Remedies. New Canaan, CT: Keats, 1979.

Bear, Jessica, N.D. Practical Uses and Applications of the Bach Flower Emotional Remedies. Las Vegas, NV: Balancing Essentials Press, 1993.

Kaminski, Patricia and Richard Katz. Flower Essence Repertory. Nevada City, CA: Flower Essence Society, 1994.

Kaslof, Leslie J. The Bach Remedies: A Self-Help Guide. New Canaan, CT: Keats, 1988.

Petrak, Joyce. How to Remember Bach Flower Remedies. Warren, MI: Curry-Peterson Press, 1992.

Scheffer, Mechtild. Bach Flower Therapy. Rochester, VT: Inner Traditions, 1987.

Weeks, Nora and Victor Bullen. The Bach Flower Remedies. London: C.W. Daniel Company, 1973.

SELF MASSAGE INSTRUCTIONAL GUIDES

Carter, Mildred. Body Reflexology. W. Nyack, NY: Parker Publishing, 1994.

Cerney, J.V. Acupuncture Without Needles. W. Nyack, NY: Parker Publishing, 1983.

Gach, Michael R. Acupressure's Potent Points. New York: Bantam Books, 1990.

Kushi, Michio. Book of Do-In. Tokyo: Japan Publications, 1995.

RECIPES GALORE

Abehsera, Michel. Cooking with Care & Purpose. Brooklyn, NY: Swan House Publishers, 1978.

Balch, James, M.D. Dietary Wellness. Greenfield, Indiana: PAB Publishing, 1993.

Brody, Jane. Good Food Book. New York: Bantam, 1987.

Colbin, Anne Marie. Book of Whole Meals. New York: Ballantine Books, 1985.

Mackenzie, Shea. The Garden of Earthly Delights Cookbook. Garden City, NY: Avery, 1993.

Ornish, Dean, M.D. Everyday Cooking with Dr. Dean Ornish. New York: HarperCollins, 1996.

Raichlen, Steven. High-Flavor, Low-Fat Vegetarian Cooking. New York: Viking, 1995.

Saltzman, Joanne. Amazing Grains. Tiburon, CA: HJ Kramer, 1990.

Vegetarian Times Complete Cookbook. New York: Macmillan, 1995.

OUR OWN REFERENCE LIBRARY

Balch, James F., M.D. and Phyllis A. Balch, C.N.C. Prescription for Nutritional Healing. New York: Avery Publishing, 1990.

Ballantine, Rudolph, M.D. Diet & Nutrition. Honesdale, PA: Himalayan International Institute, 1978.

Colbin, Anne Marie. Food and Healing. New York: Ballantine, 1986.

Ornish, Dean, M.D. Eat More Weigh Less. New York: HarperCollins, 1993.

Reid, Daniel. The Complete Book of Chinese Health and Healing. Boston: Shambhala, 1994.

Robbins, John. May All Be Fed—Diet for a New World. New York: Avon Books, 1992.

Robbins, John. Diet For a New America. Walpole, NH: Stillpoint Publishing, 1993.

Shealy, Norman, M.D. and Caroline Myss. The Creation of Health. Walpole, NH: Stillpoint Publishing, 1993.

Tierra, Michael, C.A., N.D. Planetary Herbology. Sante Fe, NM: Lotus Press, 1988.

Weil, Andrew, M.D. Spontaneous Healing. New York: Alfred A. Knopf, 1995.

OUR FAVORITE MAIL ORDER SOURCES

Herbs and VitaminsEast West Products, Ltd.
P.O. Box 1210
New York, New York 10025
(212) 864-1342
Bulk herbs available in small quantities

Frontier Cooperative Herbs
P.O. Box 299
Norway, Iowa 52318
(319) 227-7991
Herbs, spices

Eclectic Institute
14385 Southeast Lusted Road
Sandy, Oregon 97055
(800) 332-4372
Freeze-dried herbal glycerine extracts, vitamins, minerals

The Vitamin Shoppe
4700 Westside Avenue
North Bergen, New Jersey 07047
(800) 223-1216

L&H Vitamins
37-10 Crescent Street
Long Island City, New York 11101
(800) 221-1152

Hickey's
888 Second Avenue
New York, New York 10017
(800) 724-5566

Foods
Mountain Ark
P.O. Box 487
Asheville, North Carolina 28802
(800) 643-8909
Vegetables, miso, seasonings, rice, pasta, fruit, spreads, oils, beans, soup

Jaffe Bros. Natural Foods
Valley Center, California 92082
(619) 749-1133
Bulk organic natural foods.

Country Store, Paul's Grains
2475-B 340th Street
Laurel, Iowa 50141
(515) 476-3373
Organically grown grains, flours, and cereals

Deer Valley Farm
R.D. 1
Guilford, New York 13780
(607) 764-8556
Natural whole food products, organic meats, Icelandic fish

Neshaminy Valley Natural Foods
421 Pike Road
Huntingdon Valley, Pennsylvania 19006
(215) 364-8440
Buying clubs of six households or more can order products

Diamond Organics
P.O. Box 2159
Freedom, California 95019
(800) 922-2396
Organic produce harvested the day of the order;
    fresh pasta, breads, olive oils, and condiments

Eden Acres, Inc.
12100 Lima Center Road
Clinton, Michigan 49235
(517) 456-4288
Organic produce

Mothers & Others for a Livable Planet
40 West 20th Street
New York, New York 10011
(212) 242-0010
Organic produce

Rising Sun Distributors
P.O. Box 627
Milesburg, Pennsylvania 16853
(814) 355-9850
Beef, poultry, lamb, pork, fruits, vegetables, beans, seeds,
    grains

Flower Essences
HQ HealthQuest, Inc.
P.O. Box 8723
Red Bank, New Jersey 07701
Toll Free: (888) 222-8400

Ellon, USA
644 Merrick Road
Lynbrook, New York 11563
(800) 434-0449

If you would like information on our FEELING LIGHT
seminars, lectures, newsletter, videotapes, audiotapes, and
nutritional products, please write or call:

> HQ HealthQuest, Inc.
> P.O. Box 8723
> Red Bank, New Jersey 07701
> Toll Free: (888) 222-8400

INDEX